# IN
# SEARCH
# OF
# GIANTS

# IN
# SEARCH
# OF
# GIANTS

**THE QUEST
TO FIND THE
GENETIC
GIANTS
OF NORTHERN
IRELAND**

## COLLEEN SNYDER
## AND BRENDAN HOLLAND

FP
FAIRSING

Library of Congress Control Number: 2024912399

Publisher's Cataloging-in-Publication Data
Names: Snyder, Colleen Grimmel, 1956- author. | Holland, Brendan Charles, 1952- author.
Title: In search of giants : the quest to find the genetic giants of Northern Ireland / Colleen Snyder and Brendan Holland.
Description: [Linden, Virginia] : Fairsing Publishing, [2024] | Includes bibliographical references.
Identifiers: ISBN: 979-8-9903015-0-4 (hardcover) | 979-8-9903015-1-1 (paperback) | 979-8-9903015-2-8 (ebook) | 979-8-9903015-3-5 (audiobook) | LCCN: 2024912399
Subjects: LCSH: Holland, Brendan Charles, 1952- | Snyder, Colleen Grimmel, 1956- | Gigantism-- Patients--History. | Gigantism--Endocrine aspects. | Gigantism--Northern Ireland. | Gigantism-- History. | Genomics. | Human genetics. | Mutation (Biology) | Endocrine genetics. | Heredity, Human. | BISAC: HEALTH & FITNESS / Diseases & Conditions / Endocrine System. | SCIENCE / Life Sciences / Genetics & Genomics. | BIOGRAPHY & AUTOBIOGRAPHY / Medical (incl. Patients)
Classification: LCC: RB140.5 .S69 2024 | DDC: 616.13--dc23

Names: Snyder, Colleen, author | Holland, Brendan, author.
Title: In Search of Giants: The Quest to find the Genetic Giants of Northern Ireland / Colleen Snyder and Brendan Holland.

979-8-9903015-0-4 (Hardcover)
979-8-9903015-1-1 (Paperback)

Front Cover and Book Design by theBookDesigners
Northern Ireland Map Illustration by Wren Snyder

For more information, to book an event, or to contact the authors, please go to our website www.insearchofgiants.org.

Fairsing Publishing
Linden, Virginia

FP

FAIRSING

*To my family and friends, especially my sister Cherie,*
*who have supported me along my Irish genetic journey.*

—**C S**

*To my wife Patricia, the extended Holland family, and my friends*
*at the Killeeshil & Clonaneese Historical Society who have*
*helped me in the work I've undertaken on Márta's behalf.*

—**B H**

# CONTENTS

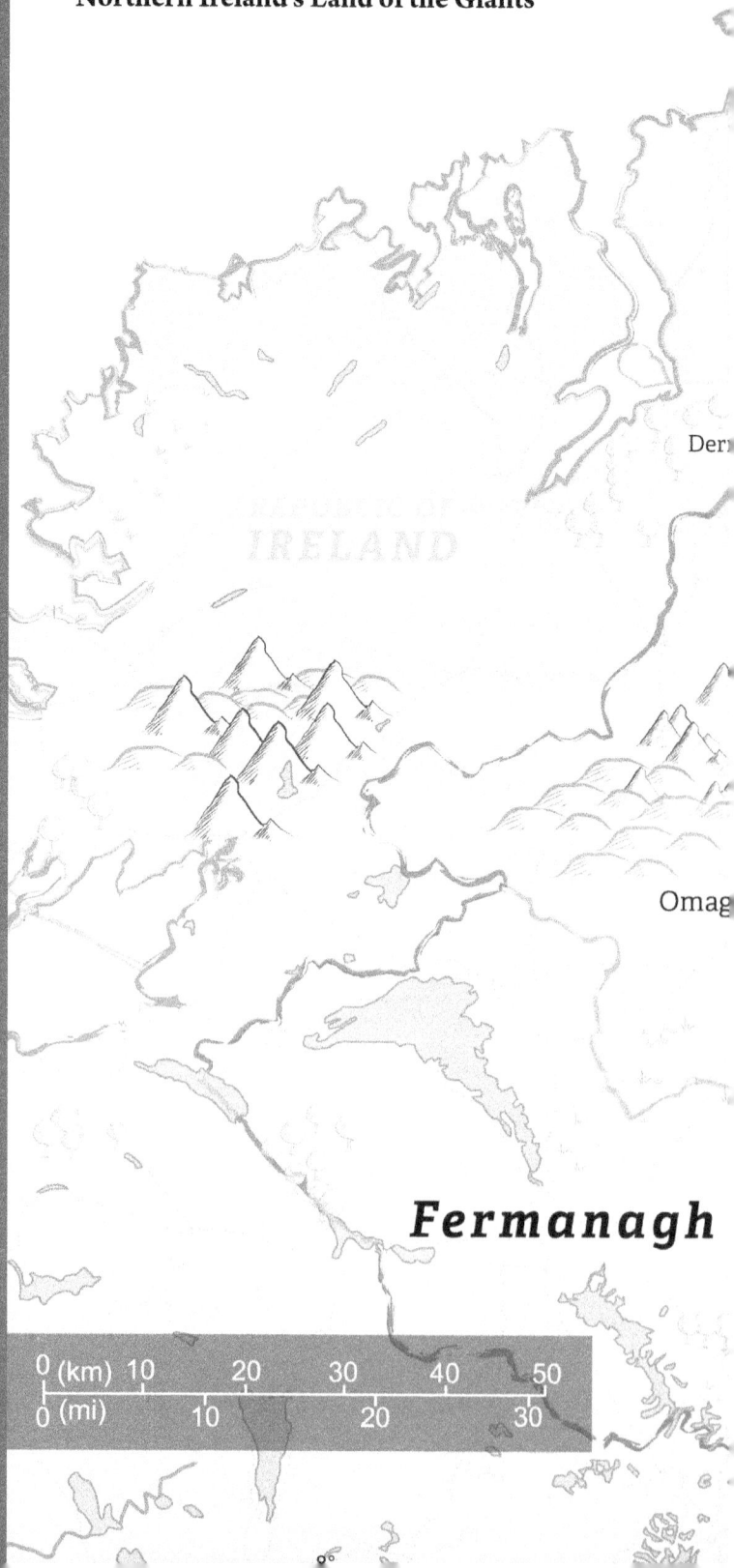

Der

REPUBLIC OF
IRELAND

Omag

*Fermanagh*

| 0 (km) 10 | 20 | 30 | 40 | 50 |
| 0 (mi) | 10 | 20 | 30 |

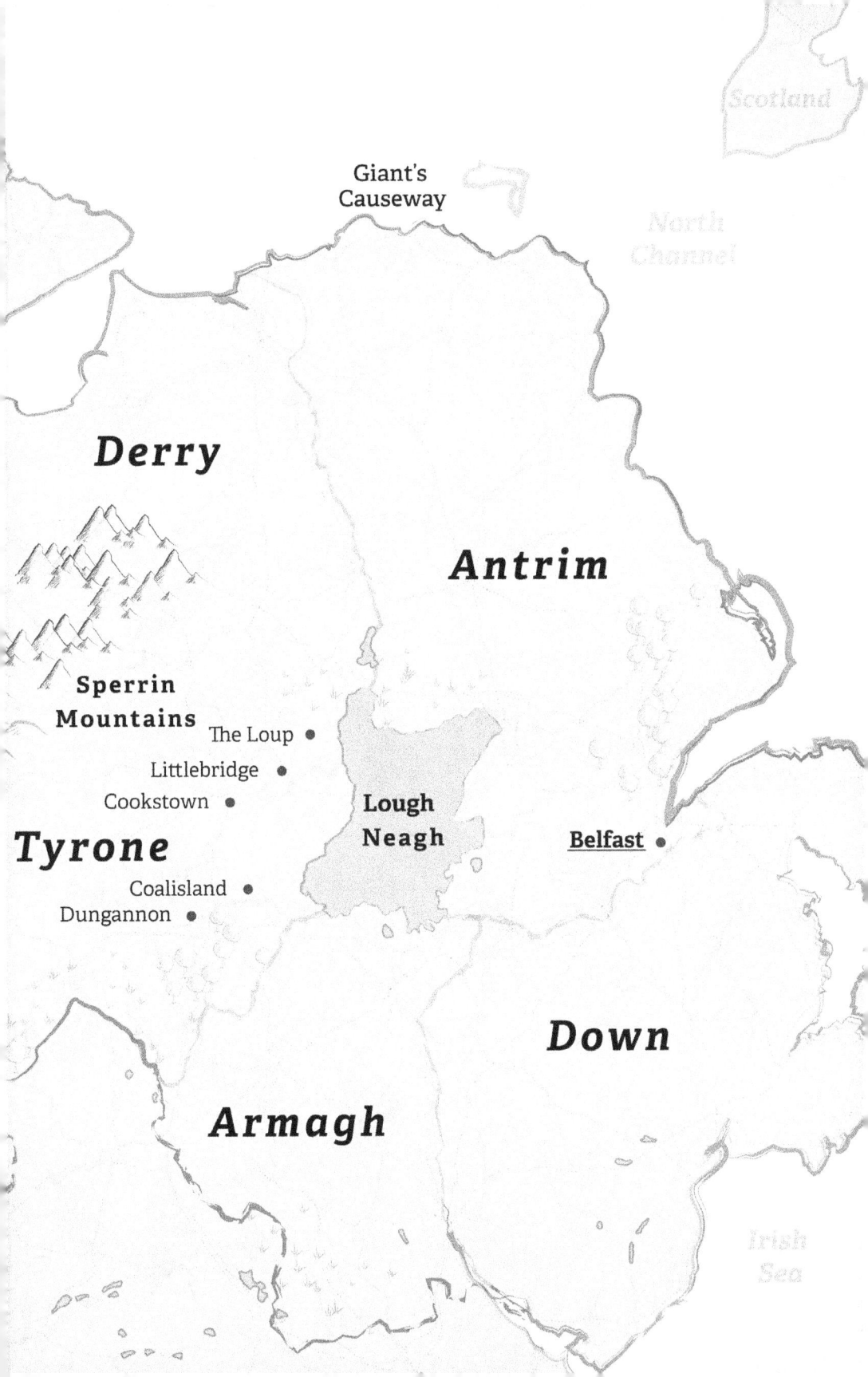

Scotland

North
Channel

Giant's
Causeway

**Derry**

**Antrim**

Sperrin
Mountains
The Loup •
Littlebridge •
Cookstown •

Lough
Neagh

Belfast •

**Tyrone**

Coalisland •
Dungannon •

**Down**

**Armagh**

Irish
Sea

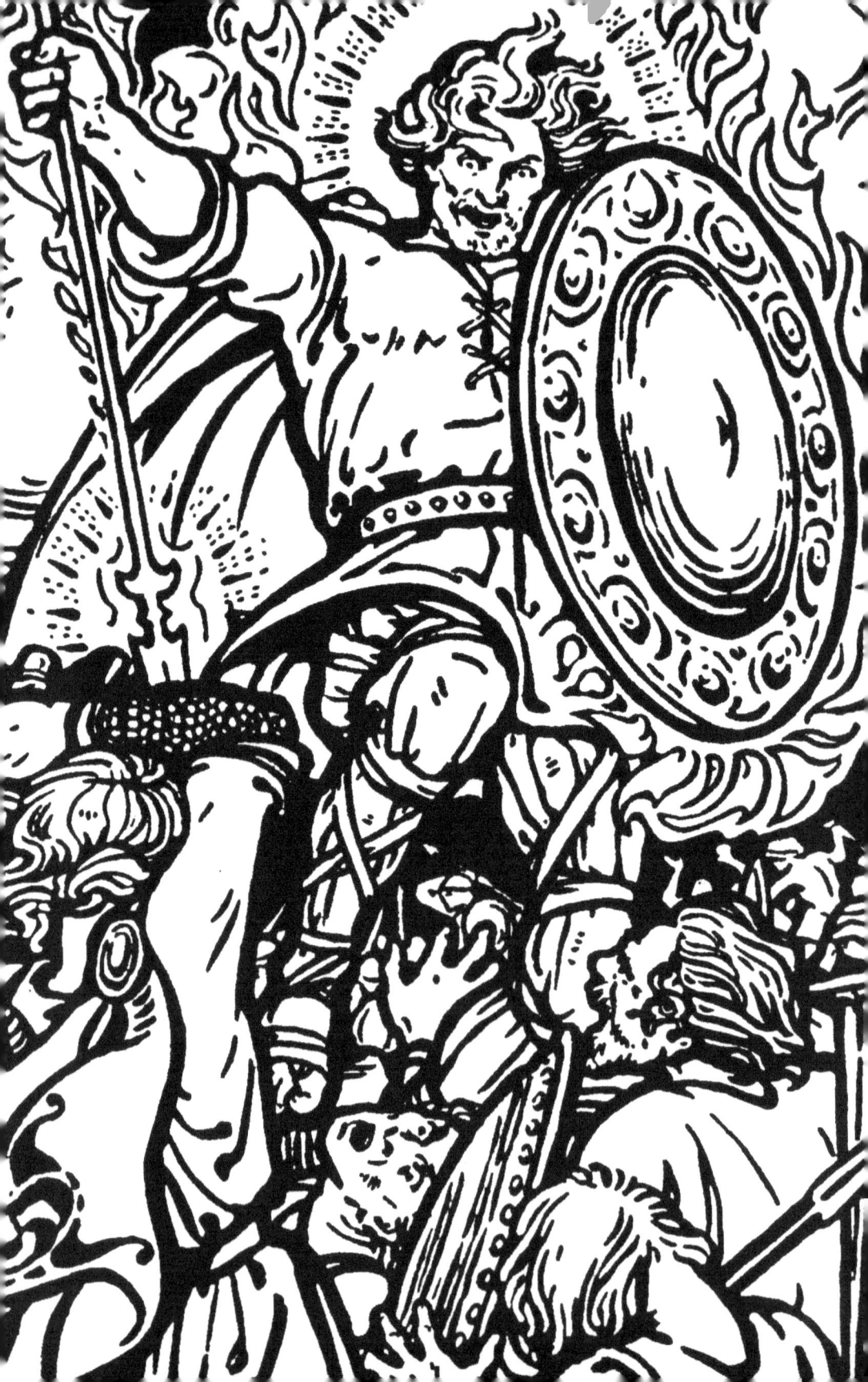

Fionn Mac Cumhaill

*Heroes of the Dawn, 1914*

"And as the foemen gazed on Fionn dread filled their hearts, for round his head shone the red light of battle, and now and again a form like a fiery serpent reared and twisted about him."

# PREFACE

As I was making my way one day in late 1972 to St. Bartholomew's Hospital in London for a medical appointment in endocrinology, a quick-witted cockney shouted at me across the street, "Oi mate, you cast a long shadow, don't you?" I smiled at him and acknowledged his wit and originality by waving back at him. I found his remark entertaining, original and funny, unlike the usual, "Aye, is it cold up there?" followed by a guffaw of laughter or the open-mouthed staring with a nudge and a comment, "God, look at that man. He's a fierce height." This is life in public when you stand out from the crowd—quite literally that is—at 6 feet, 9 inches (206 cm) tall.

In the course of a lifetime, I have met many people, but few have made the huge impact on my life and well-being as the person I was going to meet that day at St. Bartholomew's Hospital (also known as Barts), one of the finest medical institutions in the world. His name is Professor Mike Besser, and over the next three months, he oversaw my diagnosis and very successful treatment for the potentially fatal condition known as gigantism. I have often reflected how fortunate I was to meet Professor Besser, a pioneer in endocrinology and a man for whom I developed a lifelong admiration and friendship. His place in the list of great doctors of this and the last century is already assured.

Since my diagnosis and treatment in 1972, it always bugged me as to why, as one of eight siblings, I was the only one with this unusual condition. It took thirty-eight years until I learned that a genetic mutation found in my community in County Tyrone caused my gigantism. Professor Márta Korbonits, Professor Besser's protégé and successor, and her team of researchers at Barts discovered the genetic mutation in 2009. I was fortunate to meet Professor Korbonits in London to discuss the genetics behind my medical condition in 2010. She is another trailblazer in research and treatment in the field of endocrinology to the benefit of the patients who have found their way to her at Barts. When I first met her, I was drawn to her direct personality and her enthusiasm to further investigate gigantism's origins and how common it is in County Tyrone. Over the years since then, I am proud to say that Márta has become one of my closest friends.

In 2013, Márta decided to bring a global team of researchers to County Tyrone to screen the local population for the genetic mutation that can cause gigantism. She hoped to understand what percentage of the population had the genetic mutation. When she asked me to help with her research by assisting with the logistics of the population screening in County Tyrone, I was only too happy to oblige. My task was to enlist local volunteers and obtain a space for the team of endocrinologists to conduct the screening. I embarked on this project that both fascinated and intrigued me. Luckily, I had the local knowledge, both historic and geographic, that proved useful. The screening was very successful.

After the screening, it occurred to me that, given the high level of emigration from our area during and after the Great Famine of the 1840s to other countries such as the United States, Canada, and Australia, there had to be descendants of those emigrants who inherited the condition and who may well be undiagnosed and living outside of Ireland. And so, it emerged that Márta introduced me to this book's writer, Colleen Snyder, who lives in Virginia in the United States and whose ancestors once lived in County Tyrone.

Since then, Colleen and I have established a firm and lasting friendship, primarily due to our common diagnosis of gigantism. As we exchanged phone calls and talks on Zoom, we got to know more about each other and our interests. Colleen is an accomplished writer, so it became obvious to me that we should collaborate on the production of a book to include my interest in history, which was something Márta had been urging me to do. Colleen and I pooled our knowledge to increase public awareness and thereby identify potential patients who may have inherited the rogue gene that can lead to gigantism.

The world of someone with gigantism can be a lonely place, but it need not be if there is more awareness and knowledge of the problems that often come with it. I appreciate in ways that mere words cannot adequately express, the great fortune I had in meeting physicians and researchers who have contributed so much to our knowledge and understanding of my condition. This book is a tribute to their dedication and commitment to eliminating gigantism in the future.

—*Brendan Holland*
Dungannon, Northern Ireland, UK

# AUTHOR'S NOTE

A s the world shut down at the onset of the Covid-19 pandemic, my world shrank down to the pinpoint of my immediate family in my mountain home in Virginia. Like many others who found a world outside the trusted bubble of their family through their computers, I spent quite a bit of time on the internet. The computer monitor was my link to the outside world, a safe place when the broader world was so frightening during a global health crisis and a way to travel the world without leaving my office. I had no idea how much my life would change after an isolated and boring afternoon when I did a Google search about a rare disease I had as a child. I always thought that the disease was called childhood onset acromegaly. Instead, I discovered it was called gigantism.

Despite being 65 years old, I never met another person with gigantism until I met Brendan in January 2021 because of that Google search. I had no idea about the depth of giant legend and lore in Northern Ireland between Lough Neagh and the Sperrin Mountains in a geographic area known for a genetic mutation that can cause gigantism. I knew nothing about my Irish ancestors from County Tyrone who left during the Great Famine and joined the Irish diaspora in 1861, bringing a rare genetic mutation with them. I didn't know about the genetic research that led to the discovery of the genetic mutation that had so impacted my life. I had a lot to learn.

Despite living an ocean apart, Brendan and I decided to work together on the book you are about to read. Brendan became my teacher, historian, and friend to help me understand the culture, history, and language of an

Ireland I never knew. He taught me about his deep family roots in Mid-Ulster in County Tyrone, his life as a giant in Northern Ireland, and his historical research into local giant lore and legend.

My role in this book is to be the writer and tell not just our story but also the stories of others, particularly in Brendan's family, who have been affected by gigantism—a life-threatening medical condition that causes debilitating headaches, blindness, heart arrythmias, joint pain, and infertility. Because I am the writer, this book is written in American English. The quotations follow the conventions and spellings of the speaker, so you may see some British spelling along the way. I hope that this book reaches an international audience, so I also include metric measurements.

This book is about giants. Some of the giants in this book are quite tall, others are not. They have all been deeply affected by their gigantism. I hope that by the end of this book you will understand why gigantism is not just about being tall.

—*Colleen Snyder*
Linden, Virginia, US

# CHAPTER 1

# THE GIANTS AMONG US

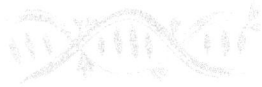

G iants loom large in our imaginations. They stand tall as objects of curiosity and wonder, but also of fear. Superhuman, they tower over the mere mortals around them. Giants fascinate and draw us towards them as we gaze up at them in awe.

Mythology and legends cast giants as capricious, malevolent, and powerful. They triumph over the world around them through their strength and stature. In Hesiod's tales of Greek mythology, the single-eyed, Cyclopes giants use their enormous strength to do battle against the Titans. They forge Zeus' mighty thunderbolt and Poseidon's deadly trident. Homer's man-eating Cyclops Polyphemus attacks Odysseus only to be blinded when Odysseus pierces his massive eye.

Norse mythology thrills with its tales of the Frost Giants who rise from primordial chaos to encase the world in ice and snow. The Norse Fire Giants bring light yet threaten to destroy the world through their fire. In the Hebrew Bible, the Nephilim, a race of giant demons representing darkness, terrify the living only to die in the floods that covered the earth in Noah's time.

Giants haunt our dreams and inhabit our childhood through fairy tales of ogres and monsters. Bellowing "Fee-fi-fo-fum," the giant of "Jack and the Beanstalk" searches for his victims to grind their bones to make his bread in one tale dating back to the early 1700s. The Brothers Grimm fairy tale "The Valiant Little Tailor" features a clever tailor who uses his wits to trick giants into believing he is stronger and braver. This leads to fame and wealth for the tailor, but only if he can escape their wrath.

It's easy to believe that giants exist only in our imaginations, but the truth is they are real, and they live among us. Some of them are documented through historical accounts. For example, James Kirkland was one of the Potsdam Giants of the *Lange Kerle* of Prussia—an elite infantry regiment of "long fellows" of exceptional height. The regiment was founded in 1675 and is still active today. Some giants became famous as carnival sideshows, such as Anna Swan (1846-1888). At 7 feet 11 inches (241 cm) tall, the Canadian woman married her equally tall husband Martin Bates (known as the Kentucky Giant). Together, they toured with the W. W. Cole Circus as the world's tallest couple.

Monster giants live on the big screen and in our television sets. Known for his distorted facial features and menacing hands, Rondo Hatton terrified moviegoers in the 1940s with his portrayal of The Creeper in *The Brute Man*, the *House of Horrors*, and *The Pearl of Death*. In the 1970s, Richard Kiel became a horror icon as the malevolent Jaws in the 007 James Bond movies.

Friendlier faces are found on television and in books. The 1960s hit television show *The Munsters* lampooned traditional monster movies and family sitcoms with its suburban family of ghouls and vampires headed up by Fred Gwynne, the Frankenstein-like father, Herman Munster. Not to be outdone, Ted Cassidy was memorable as the massive butler Lurch in the TV show *Addams Family*. The 1982 book *The BFG* by Roald Dahl brings alive a 24-foot "big, friendly giant" (hence the title) who carries orphan Sophie to his cave, where he protects her from bigger and stronger giants who might gobble her up without his protection.

Other well-known giants have found a home in wrestling. André René Rousimoff, better known as Andre the Giant, began his career as a professional wrestler in 1966, drawing crowds as he toured the world, amazing fans with his agility in the ring despite weighing more than 498 pounds (225.9 kg) at the height of his career. Maurice Tillet, rumored to be the model for the ogre Shrek in the eponymous film, completed a law degree but switched to wrestling, thinking his appearance offered him opportunities for fame and fortune unavailable to him as a lawyer.

The *Guinness World Records* is further proof that giants live today. Full of medical curiosities and human anomalies, its Hall of Fame features Sultan Kösen, the world's tallest living man, who reached 8 feet 3 inches (251 cm) tall. The sensationalism of their extreme height is on full display in the Guinness record book, but what is missing are the details of how they became so tall, the negative impact on their lives, and their poor health resulting from their stature.

When Brendan and I look at these real giants, a different story emerges. What we see is someone in pain with joints that ache from the excess growth they've endured. We see their canes, walkers, and leg braces that give them the support they need to walk when their body no longer can. We wonder if they have splitting headaches, heart arrythmias, vision loss, joint pain, infertility—all common symptoms for someone with gigantism. We note the similarity of their faces—the prominent jaw, nose, and forehead—and their oversized hands and feet. When we look at them, we see ourselves. Giants are real, and they are our kin, because we have had gigantism too.

We share a common diagnosis of gigantism,[1] a medical condition that started in childhood when a tumor on our pituitary gland triggered the pituitary to secrete excess growth hormone. Considered the master gland, the pituitary affects the entire body. The right amount of growth hormone

---

1 Over time, researchers and clinicians have used different terms for the disease of gigantism, including acromegalic gigantism, acrogigantism, childhood onset acromegaly, and pituitary gigantism. Giantism is an alternative term for the disease. For this book, I will use the widely used term gigantism with diagnostic characteristics that include childhood onset of the pituitary tumor, stature greater than the height prediction of sex-adjusted mid-parental height, and physical changes and medical conditions associated with excess growth hormone.

boosts metabolism, repairs muscles, and speeds healing. Its dysregulation causes headaches, infertility, joint pain, and hormonal imbalances. Excessive growth hormone causes the body to grow beyond its bounds. Bones lengthen, skin thickens, and facial features distort. Gigantism causes lifelong damage, both physical and emotional.

Both Brendan and I discovered that we had pituitary tumors when we turned 20 years old, but our experiences were very different.

Brendan was diagnosed in 1972 while he was working in London after he went to a routine visit with a general practitioner about some back pain he was experiencing. The doctor took note of Brendan's back pain, but much to Brendan's surprise, he quickly began to question Brendan about other symptoms he was having, including headaches, fatigue, and profuse sweating. The doctor told him that he suspected that he might have an endocrine disorder without providing any more details for his suspicions. The doctor left the room briefly. When he returned, he told Brendan to go at once to London's St. Bartholomew's Hospital for an evaluation with endocrinologist Professor Besser. Alarmed, Brendan hurried to the hospital where Professor Besser arranged his assessment, diagnosed him with acromegalic giantism (Professor Besser's preferred term in lieu of gigantism), and developed his treatment plan.

Despite being 20 years old, Brendan did not go through puberty due to his pituitary tumor, so his body continued to grow unabated. He eventually became very tall, peaking at 6 feet 11 inches (211 cm). Under the United Kingdom's National Health Service, Brendan's radiotherapy treatment that eliminated his pituitary tumor and his subsequent treatment to help with the tumor's harmful effects were fully covered. He has had continuous follow up care with endocrinologists, cardiologists, and other specialists throughout his life.

I was diagnosed in 1976 when a psychiatric nurse showed me a medical textbook with three pictures of a woman with acromegaly, the same disease but with the pituitary tumor starting to grow in adulthood rather than in

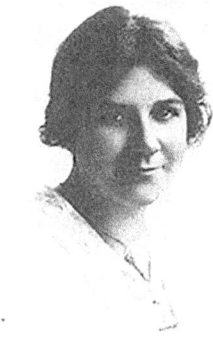

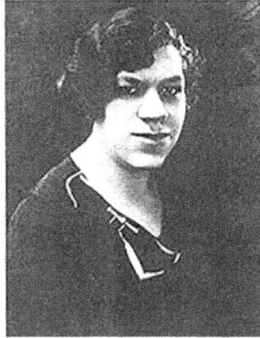

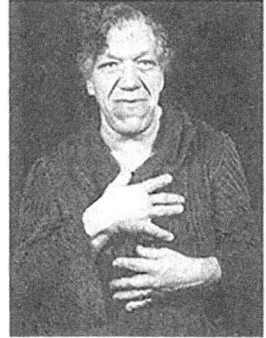

Woman with Acromegaly

childhood. The first image reveals a beautiful woman with a well-proportioned face and fine features. She looks to be about twenty years old. The second image, taken a few years later, shows how the excess growth hormone affected her face, coarsening her appearance, while the third shows her as a middle-aged woman and reveals how radically her looks uglified. I could see myself in the second picture when I looked at how her face changed as she developed a broad nose, prominent chin, and thickened skin, all characteristic markers of those with gigantism or acromegaly. I was terrified that I would eventually look like the woman in the third picture.

When I visited the endocrinologist Dr. Canary at Georgetown University Hospital to confirm the diagnosis, I brought along my school portrait photographs as he requested. At the time, I found his request curious and wondered what he wanted to do with the photographs. He placed my pictures side-by-side on his desk, one for each year from kindergarten to my senior year in high school and paused at each one to

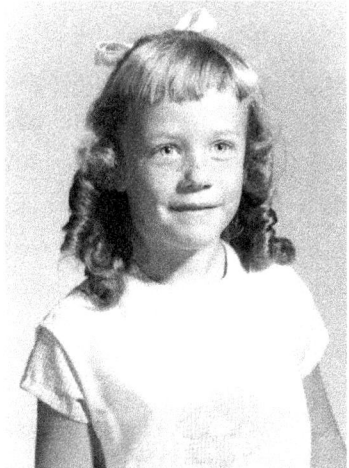

Colleen, age 5

5

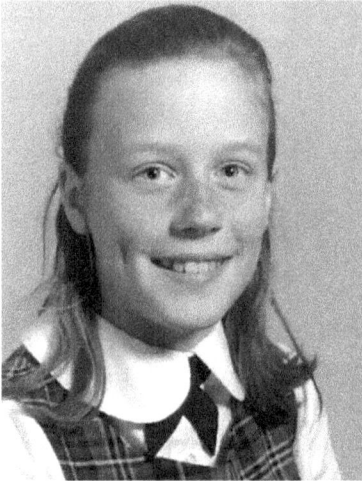

Colleen, third grade, age 9

scrutinize my face. He then looked up at me and said as he pointed to my third-grade picture, "This one. This is when you started to develop the pituitary tumor." He showed me how my face elongated from the previous year and how much my nose grew. He showed me how those changes became more pronounced year after year with the last picture from my senior year showing how dramatically different my face looked from the first picture in the array in front of him. I remembered third grade clearly because that was the year I started to go through puberty and have periods.

I found out later that how old I was when the tumor started in relation to when I began to go through puberty determined how tall I eventually became. Tumor onset and puberty are different for each person who develops gigantism. Our stature is different, but the negative impact of a dysregulated endocrine system is the same.

Before puberty, bones grow from the ends, but when puberty occurs, after a temporary yet rapid acceleration of bone growth, the bones start sealing off at their ends, limiting growth. However, when puberty is delayed, as it was in Brendan's case, the effect of excess growth hormone on bone growth is not limited by the effects of puberty, which curtails bone growth. Bones continue to grow more rapidly than normal, and excessive height occurs. Delayed puberty is often caused by the pituitary tumor itself.

In my case, my bones had just begun to seal off when I was around eight years old due to puberty, a process that takes a few years. This process dampened the effect of excess growth hormone on my bone growth. I grew to be six feet tall (183 cm), a short giant but a giant, nonetheless.

This was in stark contrast to my family with my 5 feet 2 inches (157 cm) sister and my parents who were both around 5 feet 6 (168 cm) inches.

I was lucky that successful surgery removed the tumor in 1976. However, because I was in the American healthcare system, my parents struggled to pay the medical bills. I lost my health insurance six months after the surgery when I turned 21 years old and had to go off my parent's insurance policy. Because I then had a pre-existing con-

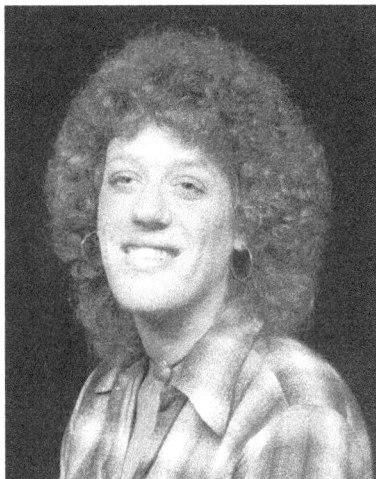

Colleen before treatment, age 20

dition, I could not find health insurance to cover my medical bills. I received little follow up care, despite the headaches, joint pain, vision loss, and menstrual problems I continued to have.

While I found out later how my experience with a pituitary tumor differed from Brendan's given how tall we became and how our healthcare was delivered, in many respects, our experiences were the same. Though small, the tumor was powerful enough to totally disrupt both of our lives, changing our faces and bodies. It was hidden, lurking throughout our childhoods, waiting until we were 20 years old to be discovered. It was relentless, continuing to damage our skeletons, even as our acromegalic features have softened now that our bodies are not being flooded with growth hormone.

Developing a pituitary tumor during childhood that results in gigantism is exceedingly rare. Pituitary tumors that cause excess growth hormone are much more common in adults, long after the person has gone through puberty. In adulthood, the disease is called acromegaly. The patients will not become abnormally tall, but they will still face all the other detrimental effects of having a pituitary tumor that causes excess growth hormone, such as vision loss, infertility, and severe headaches.

The pituitary tumor was gone; however, the damage to our bodies remained. We would feel the effect of having the tumor throughout our lives. We knew why we had the symptoms that we had that led to our diagnosis. The question of why this happened to us lingered. It would take another thirty-odd years before the field of genetics could answer that question.

After being treated for a pituitary tumor in 1976 and knowing the damage that the excess growth hormone did to my body, I wondered what the future held for me medically, and I was curious to know if others had a similar experience to mine. Most doctors I encountered knew little about acromegaly or gigantism, and they usually had never met a patient with the condition. Given its rarity, I found it extremely difficult to find any information about the long-term effects of having excess growth hormone as a child. Periodically, in hopes of finding other patients with the same disease, I reached out via endocrinology patient forums on the internet in hopes of finding someone with the disease. I found some patients with acromegaly but no one who had a pituitary tumor as a child. By the time I reached my 60s, I had all but given up hope that I would ever meet someone with the same condition. Curiosity still made me wonder why I developed this rare disease, so occasionally I typed "childhood onset acromegaly" (the term that doctors had used with me when I was diagnosed) into a search engine to see if anything new popped up in the results.

It was October 2020, and I was seven months into pandemic lockdown. It was a world in suspended animation as I watched the days slowly tick by and the death toll mount. Pandemic fatigue set in with no end in sight. I was tired of thinking about whether we had enough toilet paper or if the face masks I was sewing together from swatches of leftover fabric I scavenged from my sewing supplies would do any good. To fend off boredom, I spent one morning taking on the long-overdue chore of cleaning out our basement. By afternoon, I was ready for a break. I headed to my office and booted up my computer which would take me, at least virtually, somewhere other than my home.

Some time had passed since I last consulted "Dr. Google" about my medical mystery, so I typed "childhood acromegaly" into the search engine and idly scrolled through the results until one of them jumped out at me. It was a 2011 research paper I had never seen before with the title "*AIP* Mutation in Pituitary Adenomas in the 18th Century and Today," that used the word adenoma instead of tumor when referring to a pituitary tumor.[2] Interesting, I thought. Did *AIP* mutation mean pituitary tumors could be genetic? And what did that have to do with the 18th century? What in the world was this about?

I clicked on the link and read the article even though I didn't fully understand the technical aspects of the paper. The paper was about how London researcher Professor Márta Korbonits investigated a specific version of a genetic mutation[3] in the *AIP* gene discovered by Finnish researchers.[4] Like other *AIP* mutations, this version can cause childhood onset pituitary tumors that lead to gigantism. What was distinctive about her research, however, was how she was able to link this version to families from a small area of Northern Ireland west of Lough Neagh in Counties Tyrone and Derry and trace the history of the mutation back to the 1700s.

Now I was really drawn in, especially given that I am of Irish descent on my mother's side. However, I didn't think the research applied to me

---

2  Harvinder S. Chahal et al., "*AIP* Mutation in Pituitary Adenomas in the 18th Century and Today," *The New England Journal of Medicine* 365, no. 8 (2011).

3  A gene mutation is a change in the genome. Every gene mutation does not cause a disease. However, over time, gene mutation has come to mean a difference that causes harm. More recently, scientists use the term "gene variant" to describe a change or difference and then modify it to give information about the change in the DNA. For example, a pathogenic gene variant is used to describe a change in a gene that can lead to a disease. Very often these terms are used interchangeably depending on the context. For this book, I will be using both as well with explanations where necessary to clarify if the change in the gene can or has caused a disease.

4  Outi Vierimaa, et al. "Pituitary adenoma predisposition caused by germline mutations in the *AIP* gene." *Science*. 2006 May 26;312(5777):1228-1230.

because I remembered my mother telling me that our ancestors were from the far south of Ireland in County Cork. But then another memory popped into my head. I was back in the hospital in 1976 before I had surgery for my pituitary tumor. My mother told me that she knew a cousin on the Irish side of our family who was a Catholic priest. He stood out in her memory because he was so tall with large hands and feet. She wondered if there was any link between me and the Catholic priest. A wave of grief came over me as I thought about her and how she died in 1985. There was no way to ask her more about the priest or exactly where our ancestors once lived.

The next morning, I went back to cleaning out the basement, and by coincidence, I came across a box with family history memorabilia that I didn't remember storing. I riffled through the jumbled box with its black and white photographs of a childhood pet, an old wedding invitation, and a program from a kindergarten play I was in, when I noticed a thick, manila envelope tucked in the side of the box. It appeared unopened. I pulled it out and saw that it was postmarked 2000 and was addressed to me from my mother's brother Cecil who moved from Baltimore to Colorado in 1964. I only saw him a few times since his move and knew that he died in 2016, but I didn't remember getting the envelope.

I ripped open the envelope and pulled out a sheaf of folded papers and some photographs. To my surprise, the papers were an extensively researched family tree of the Irish side of my family, complete with details going back to the early 1800s. I found my name on the tree and traced my history back through my mother, my grandmother, my great grandfather, and stopped at my great-great grandfather John Robert McGuirk who emigrated from Ireland in 1861. I was shocked to see that he was born in County Tyrone near Coalisland, the area referenced in the research paper I read the previous day.

I grabbed the photographs to see what clues they held. As I flipped through them, I came across one of a Catholic priest labeled Father John McGuirk, again I stopped. I knew immediately it was the same person my mother mentioned. He was sitting in a red velvet, high-backed chair, high-ball in hand, looking directly into the camera. I clearly saw his elongated face, prominent jaw, large hands, and even larger feet. It was unmistakable. He had gigantism, and he was my blood relative.

I hurried up to my office to look at the article online. The pieces fell into place. First, my Irish ancestors came from the north of Ireland not the south. I had a blood relative who had gigantism. Third, I had a pituitary tumor that started in childhood. I was always proud of my Irish heritage, and I now knew that it could explain why I had this rare disease.

At first, I was stunned and just stared at the screen. Now what? What do I do with this information? I rarely talked about what I went through as a child growing up with an undiagnosed pituitary tumor. After the exhaustion of spending all of August 1976 in the hospital, I returned to college only two weeks after surgery and told no one about what happened to me. I was embarrassed and ashamed about having a tumor, so I locked the memories away. I tried to compartmentalize the experience for the rest of my life. I never discussed the full extent of my medical condition with my three children. None of my current friends knew what I went through. Both my mother and father were gone, and since my mother's death I had very limited contact with any of my relatives. I barely talked about it with my husband. I was very close to my only sister Cherie, but even she didn't know the full extent of what happened to me.

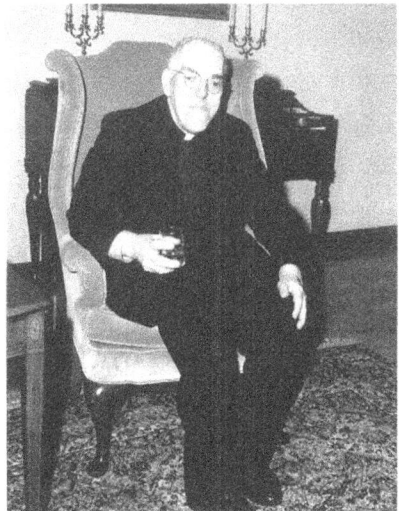

Father John McGuirk

I told my sister and my husband, but I decided to keep my suspicions about having a genetic mutation to myself and quietly figure out how

11

to get tested for the genetic mutation before telling others. I had no idea where to begin. Then I remembered that I had an endocrinology appointment set up for the following week. Maybe she could help me. I fired off an email to her with a link to the article and details about my family history. She emailed me back the next day letting me know that she instructed a company to mail me the necessary test kit, which arrived a week later. I spit into the kit's enclosed tube, sealed it up, and popped the kit back in the mail.

I tried not to think about the test, but I was eager to get the results and nervous about what it would mean if I did have the genetic mutation. Christmas and New Year's Day passed without results. Finally on January 11, 2021, I opened my email inbox and saw a message from the testing company with an attached report. I clicked on the report. I was positive for an *AIP* mutation—the same Arg304Stop mutation identified in families from Northern Ireland that I read about in the research paper.

I was thrilled, elated to finally have an answer to why I developed a pituitary tumor. But then my heart sank. What did this mean for my family and my three adult children? My older son was getting married and planning on starting a family of his own. I was alarmed that I might pass the gene on to a future grandchild. I thought of Professor Korbonits. Could she give me more information? Could she connect me with someone else with the same condition? I had to find out. I scrambled to find the research paper again, scanned down to find her email address, and tapped out a message with my diagnosis, test results, and family and medical history. I hit send not knowing if my message would even make it past her spam filter. With a sigh, I went to the kitchen to start dinner.

After dinner, I checked my tablet for messages. To my amazement, there was an answer from her in my inbox despite it being 10 pm in London. "Indeed, you have the same mutation as the Irish giants we have described." It turned out that I was the first person identified in the

United States with the Northern Ireland version of the *AIP* mutation.[5]

"I can put you in touch with Mr. Brendan Holland, who is the main person in the link I am sending you. He always told me I must find the relatives in the US as many families moved to the East Coast from that part of Northern Ireland. So pretty sure he is a cousin of yours." The link was to the 2011 BBC documentary *Charles Byrne: The Irish Giant/an Fathach Éireannach* directed by Ronan McCloskey[6] about her research, Brendan, and the famous 18th century Irish giant Charles Byrne.

I was a whirlwind of emotions: stunned that I was the first person in the US identified with the mutation; overjoyed to finally have an answer to why I had the tumor in the first place; floored to discover I had an Irish cousin Brendan; curious about Charles Byrne; eager to watch the documentary; and concerned about what this discovery meant for my family, especially my three children. I grabbed the phone and called my sister. The words tumbled out as I told her about what I discovered. I went from knowing nothing to seeing hundreds of years of family history with blood relatives stretching out before me into the distant past. I waited so long for information and now I was flooded with amazing details. In the 19th century, my great-great grandfather looked across the ocean to America to find a new life when he left Coalisland in County Tyrone. Now, in the 21st century, his great-great granddaughter was looking back to his homeland with many questions about the future for me given my genetic legacy.

A few days later, with his permission, Professor Korbonits relayed Brendan contact information to me. I was excited and extremely nervous about sending him an email, not knowing what to expect or whether he would welcome my questions. A few minutes after I hit send, I was startled when the phone rang.

---

5 The DNA sequencing performed in the US laboratory determined that I had the mutation but did not perform any other tests. However, it is extremely unlikely that the mutation was not the Northern Ireland version given my family pedigree, clear family linkage to the geographic hotspot near Cookstown in Northern Ireland, and how my DNA results corresponded with Brendan's when paired through GEDMatch.

6 *Charles Byrne: the Irish Giant/an Fathach Éireannach*, directed by Ronan McCloskey (BBC Northern Ireland, 2011), https://www.youtube.com/watch?v=xLA-KZ7sBLg.

It was Brendan. As I heard his unmistakable Irish accent when I answered the call, I was on the verge of tears. After searching for more than 45 years to find someone who could understand what I experienced, I was now talking with someone who shared my diagnosis. The catch in my voice quickly disappeared as I was swept away into our conversation. I felt that I had always known him. The kinship of our shared pituitary tumors and experiences forged an immediate friendship as we talked about how we were diagnosed, treated, and have lived with gigantism. We commiserated over splitting headaches, excessive growth, and painful joints and remembered the flood of relief when we finally had a diagnosis, both of us at age 20.

Despite our similarities, what struck me most was just how different our experiences were. He had a deep sense of his place in Irish history and a profound connection to the land around him that was steeped in legends and folklore about giants that marked Northern Ireland as a land of giants. As one of the first people that Professor Korbonits discovered to have the mutation in 2009, he was pivotal in her research to find others who either had the condition or were carriers. He had many years to think about her research and how it led to the discovery of undiagnosed individuals who went on to have timely treatment.

As a local historian, Brendan took me through centuries of local history, legends, and lore related to local giants, both from the distant past and still living. He rooted me in the land with stories about nearby places and landmarks named for giants, and he talked about local people and relatives that he knew who had gigantism, his cousin who had a stroke during the surgery to remove her tumor, and his niece who suffered from infertility prior to her treatment. He touched on how he met Professor Korbonits, how he was committed to helping her with her research when he could, and the times he talked about gigantism in documentaries, television, and radio in the search to find those with the condition and help them.

My sense of my place in history was upended. I considered myself to be of Irish descent, yet unlike Brendan, I knew little about my family history or the land of my ancestors. I realized that I had an extended family of distant cousins who share the same DNA with me and ancestors who lived hundreds, if not thousands, of years ago in Ireland. I could feel Ireland's pull, enticing me to go to the land of giants last known in my family history four generations ago when my great-great-grandfather left his home in County Tyrone to live in Baltimore.

Through video meetings, emails, and phone calls over the following months, Brendan and I became fast friends, eventually deciding to work on this book project together. He linked me to the old land through quintessential 21st-century ways to communicate. He helped me to understand Professor Korbonits' lifelong dedication to medical research, her tenacity in tracking down data about the genetic mutation, and her deep empathy for people with gigantism. I learned how one small genetic mutation can lead to lifelong changes and medical challenges. I learned that according to the medical definition of gigantism, being a giant was not just about being extremely tall. I learned giants are real, and I am a part of that community.

As we continued to meet online, Brendan told me stories of local landmarks such as the Giant's Grave in the Sperrin Mountains and the limestone quarry near Cookstown where an ordnance survey recorded the discovery of giant human bones. He referred me to mythology and folklore related to giants and the land they inhabited. He explained how Jonathan Swift wrote parts of his famous *Gulliver's Travels* while staying at Loughry Manor not far from the limestone quarry, and how Swift must have been aware of the giant legends so popular in the area and had possibly met living giants who resided in the geographic hotspot. I knew that meeting Brendan over the internet was only the beginning of my journey.

As I heard Brendan's stories, I was awestruck by the mythical Irish giants of the north. I immersed myself in fabulous tales of days long ago when giants held sway over the land with the strength to destroy and reshape it or the compassion to build and protect it. I began to understand how deeply the roots of gigantism ran in Mid-Ulster Northern Ireland bounded by the Sperrin Mountains to the west and Lough Neagh to the east. I realized that my roots were in that geographic hotspot, and I wanted to know how my one small branch connected to those roots.

The more I learned about my ancestral home, the more I wanted to go to the land of giants to make a tangible connection with Brendan and visit where my great-great grandfather lived before he left Ireland to find his new home in America. I called up my travel-loving sister and pitched a trip to Northern Ireland. I told her how much I wanted to go there and hoped that she would be just as interested. It wasn't a hard sell. She didn't hesitate; she was in. We didn't know when we made our pact to travel to Northern Ireland that the pandemic would drag on, and it would be 18 long months before the lockdown eased and we felt safe enough to travel.

# CHAPTER 2

# A LIFE REFLECTED

T alking with Brendan over the months in lockdown was a welcome respite from the pandemic. I found it fascinating to do research on the stories he told me about local giants whenever boredom crept in. I'd flip on my computer, leave my pandemic world behind, and wander the internet looking for details about the giants I encountered in Brendan's stories.

Because I never knew anyone with a pituitary tumor, I was naturally curious to hear all the details about how Brendan was diagnosed and treated, and I was eager to hear about any psychological and physical challenges that we might share. I was also intrigued by his rural life in Northern Ireland.

Brendan was generous and kind in sharing his story with me whenever we met on Zoom. I enjoyed hearing about his childhood, which was so different from mine growing up in the suburbs of Washington, DC. He recounted his earliest memories of growing up in rural Ackinduff, just eight miles west of Dungannon in County Tyrone. He told me that he was born at home in 1952 into a large family with seven siblings that

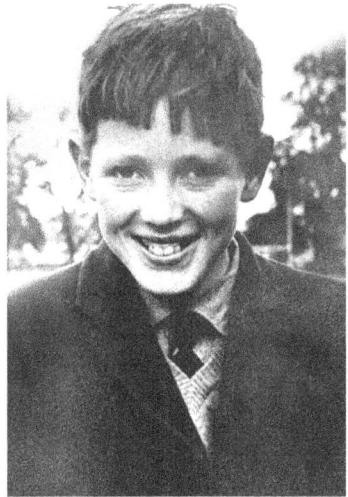

Brendan, age 12

gave him a "sense of complete security and love" and as the second youngest in the family, he knew that he was "a member of a close family group who were always encouraged to look after each other."

Brendan emphasized that the security that he still holds so dear came not only from his immediate family but also from the extended clan of Hollands who lived close to him. The four other Holland families in Ackinduff rooted him deeply in his rural community as he grew up in the 1950s and 1960s in Northern Ireland. He told me that they were "close as all our parents were good friends who shared their workload when harvest time came around. The cutting of hay, gathering of potatoes, the cutting of turf in the bog for winter fuel, the harvesting of the barley and corn were all times of the year when we intermingled freely and happily without a care in the world." As the Hollands walked down the winding dirt road lined with blackthorn hedgerows to Mass, it was a time to socialize, tell stories, and enjoy each other's company. He emphasized how wonderful his memories were of that simpler time, making "no apology for portraying this experience as an ideal childhood because that is what it was."

But as he grew to be nearly six feet tall (183 cm) and entered his teenage years, a darker side of the broader community outside the loving embrace of the Holland clan came into focus. At first, he enjoyed being taller than his fellow classmates; however, as he grew, the hurtful comments from the other teenagers became more frequent. "As my height increased to unusual levels, I became more self-conscious. I remember that feeling and the unwelcome barbs, by children especially, when I was called a monster and other such insults. These comments played on my mind and made me more self-conscious about my height. As a consequence, I became even more introverted."

For Brendan, the psychological and physical effects of the disease took their greatest toll when he had to give up his cherished sport of Gaelic football.[1]

---

1 Gaelic football is a popular amateur sport in Ireland that is similar to a combination of soccer and rugby. The sport is governed by the Gaelic Athletic Association (GAA) and holds significant cultural and historical importance in Irish society.

"In my first year of St. Patrick's Academy grammar school, I was selected for the third-year Gaelic football team because at that time I was a decent player. All that was to change in a short time as I lost my stamina, coordination, and speed—all necessary attributes for this wonderful sport. I just couldn't understand it at the time. In hindsight, this was at a time when my production of growth hormone was at its zenith, and my metabolic system was in a poor state. I now recognize that one's lowest ebb, physically, can also be the same, psychologically."

As Brendan neared the end of his schooling, he became even more introverted as he became increasingly aware of how different his body was from his peers. "In my late teens up until the diagnosis of my illness, I stopped socializing as much as I normally did as I was becoming increasingly conscious of my height and how it made me stand out from the crowd. I noticed that, unlike my contemporaries, I had not begun to shave, and I perspired profusely. Some of my more mean-minded friends also noticed and took every opportunity to remind me of my shortcomings."

While I had the difficulty of going through puberty when I was only eight years old, Brendan had an equally complicated challenge of not going through puberty until after he was treated for his pituitary tumor. There is nothing unusual about teenagers being focused on their bodies and making comments about others. Teenagers are normally very aware and self-conscious of the changes that puberty brings. However, for people with gigantism, the teenage years can be particularly horrific, as excess growth hormone and other hormones affected by the pituitary tumor distort the body to a greater degree than normal puberty. In addition, going through puberty triggers the body to stop growing, which did not happen in Brendan's case.

Body image suffers severely. Brendan vividly remembers the confusion he felt. "Even though I was suffering from severe headaches and excess tiredness for most of the time I had not managed to join up the dots, so to speak. None of this made any sense to me but in the back of my mind

I began to wonder if something was very wrong with me. Was it physical, was it psychological, or was I just being overly sensitive?"

As I got to know more about his life growing up in Northern Ireland in the 1960s, it seemed inevitable that our discussions included the political turmoil of the Troubles[2] going on at that time. Brendan reminded me that the Troubles actually started in Dungannon in August 1968, when Northern Ireland's first civil rights protesters marched from Coalisland to Dungannon only to clash with loyalist counter-protesters. While his values were being challenged by the activities of extremist groups on both sides of his community, Brendan felt he was fortunate to be at St. Patrick's Academy grammar school where teachers encouraged discussions about the significance of the violent upheaval. These discussions "fired my interest in history as the causes of these events lay there and in the previous centuries of Ireland's troubled past." Just as the community of Northern Ireland itself was going through so much systemic pain, so was Brendan as he experienced the disturbing physical changes and pain he felt throughout his body.

By the time Brendan turned 17 in 1969, his symptoms accelerated. He shot up more than four inches to 6 feet 4 inches (193 cm). His fatigue increased, and his headaches grew even more painful. He told me about one terrifying episode. "I was in the classroom during a French lesson, copying material from the blackboard when I blacked out. I could not see anything, and I had a very violent headache." When his parents found out what happened, they took him to their family doctor who referred him to the Dungannon hospital. He was admitted for a week of testing and examinations, only to be discharged without any reason given for his symptoms. "That is where it ended as there was no discussion with me or my parents as to the nature of my diagnosis or even that I had a serious medical condition."

---

2 The Troubles in Northern Ireland was a period of bloody sectarian violence between mostly Catholic nationalists, who wanted to join Ireland, and mostly Protestant unionists, who wanted to stay part of the United Kingdom. It lasted about 30 years and ended with the Good Friday peace agreement in 1998.

"It was at this time that my extraordinary height began to bother me. Local people, I felt, made a big issue about it, which only served to increase my self-consciousness. I also knew I was different than my contemporaries in appearance due to my lack of physical maturity. It made me more introverted and uncertain of my personal identity. In short, my self-confidence was plummeting."

Two years later, in 1971, Brendan decided to move to London rather than remain in the Dungannon area after graduation. "I felt that I could lose myself in the big crowd of a city as opposed to standing out in the more parochial society of Dungannon." By now, his height was well outside the norm as he grew another four inches, measuring in at 6 feet 10 inches (193 cm).

He found a temporary job at the Maudsley Hospital in Camberwell, South London, in the medical records department for several mental health outpatient clinics. The job was an eye-opener. "These clinics covered the whole gambit of mental health issues and opened a whole new area of the human condition that I had not been exposed to in my rural upbringing. I was amazed by this new experience." One patient stood out. "I was most interested in patients with sexual identity problems. One young man was preparing to have a sex change operation. He had gender issues from an early age. When he reached adulthood, he left home in rural England and came to London so he could get lost in the anonymity of the big city. This struck a chord with me. I could sympathize with his predicament." His story about the patients in the clinic with sexual identity issues resonated with me as well because I remembered how I questioned my own sexual identity before I had surgery. The hormonal dysregulation from having a pituitary tumor caused my voice to deepen and my shoulders to widen, making me look and sound quite masculine, which I found very disturbing.

As his job in the mental health department came to an end, and he moved on to work at two short term jobs simultaneously, Brendan struggled. "I was permanently tired, had constant throbbing headaches, and a nagging worry that I was still only shaving very irregularly." Things came to a head in early April 1972. Brendan woke up with severe pain in his back. "Given I was working two jobs, I felt that perhaps I was overdoing things, and that my body was confirming it. I also felt generally unwell. These concerns gnawed at my mind for some time, and I decided to do something about it." He was able to get a same-day appointment for 10:00 am at his local doctor's office.

When Brendan told the doctor about his backache, he was taken aback and concerned when the doctor's questions quickly turned to other problems that Brendan mentioned. "I explained my backache as best I could, but he seemed more interested in my other problems, particularly the lack of facial hair and my throbbing headaches. His probing questions began to concern and upset me, and I could feel tears well up in my eyes. This was beginning to frighten me as I had been conscious for some time of my still boyish features, which were out of keeping with a 20-year-old youth who was almost seven feet tall (213 cm)."

Brendan's concerns grew as the doctor stepped out of the office to make a phone call after completing his examination. When the doctor returned, Brendan's world turned upside down. Brendan remembers how disoriented he felt as the realization that he had a serious medical condition swept over him. "The doctor told me that he thought I had a serious glandular condition and that he wanted me to go immediately to St. Bartholomew's Hospital to see an endocrinology specialist at 2:30 pm the same day. My mind was racing between concerns about informing my boss that I couldn't be at work and wondering why there was such a rush. I was so overcome that I neglected to ask him that obvious question. It was only when I was on my way back to my bedsit that I realized the seriousness of my situation. I was probably going to be the subject of an intense examination of both body and mind."

When Brendan arrived at the outpatient department at St. Bartholomew's Hospital, he only waited a few minutes before he heard a deep voice call his name, and Professor Mike Besser, one of the top endocrinologists in the United Kingdom, entered his life. "This impressive doctor exuded an air of confidence, and I somehow felt comfortable in his presence. He spoke with authority but not arrogance, even when he spoke to his junior colleagues. There were at least six white-coat-clad doctors accompanying Professor Besser, but there was no doubt about who was in charge."

Brendan remembered the depth of the medical examination and the extreme emotions that he felt. "I distinctly recall feeling extremely nervous and hypersensitive—so much so that I could feel the perspiration running down each side of my torso from my armpits. What, in God's name, had I let myself in for? Only a few hours earlier, I decided to visit my doctor and here I was, in a room full of curious young doctors. Then the questions started, and they became more and more personal." The doctors quizzed him on his headaches, his delayed puberty, and his lack of facial and body hair. They conducted a full physical examination, "so that I ended up on a bed with nothing on other than my birthday suit with the salty sting of perspiration in my eyes."

The room emptied, except for Professor Besser. As Brendan got dressed, Professor Besser sympathetically detailed what they found. "He explained that I had a metabolic condition that was causing me to grow so tall. Most probably, I had a small tumor on my pituitary gland, which was located at the center of the skull, behind my eyes. He told me that my optic nerves were being pressurized from underneath by the tumor and that my peripheral vision was reduced. Left untreated, I would be in danger of losing my vision as the tumor could sever the optic nerves. He assured me that would not happen in the near future and that, when they completed a battery of tests, they could establish the extent of the tumor and treat it by surgery or radiation, or a combination of both." Professor Besser told Brendan that he wanted to admit him later in the week and to be prepared to be in the hospital for at least two months to allow the medical staff to complete the extensive testing needed to determine the best course of treatment to fight his pituitary tumor.

Professor Besser assured Brendan that he would make a full recovery, excused himself, and left the room. Brendan was shaken yet relieved. "I was left alone in the room, and I recall that I was extremely thirsty – no wonder, as I must have been dehydrated from the excessive perspiration. I filled a plastic cup of water, gulped it down and sat down again. Then I began to weep uncontrollably and grabbed some paper tissues to dry my eyes. So, this is the answer to those nagging worries, the bouts of extreme tiredness and the explanation for the headaches that dogged me from the age of fourteen. But I soon composed myself when I realized that I was

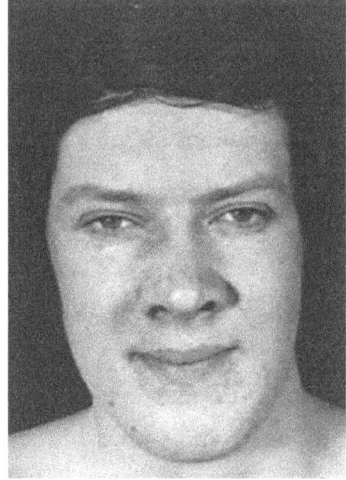

Brendan before radiotherapy, age 20

now in a good place to have something done about it, and, most importantly, Professor Besser would be there to help me."

Only 20 years old, far from home, and overwhelmed by the diagnosis, Brendan suddenly remembered that his brother Noel was in London undergoing training at the police center. The love and support so important to him in Ackinduff was only a phone call away when he reached out to his brother who rushed to his aid. "Of course, I began to get emotional but, as a policeman, he was trained to handle situations such as this. He calmed me, and in his usual systematic manner, he went through the conversation I had with Professor Besser, point by point. He told me not to worry about contacting my other brothers and sisters or Mum and Dad, which made it easier to talk to them later about this strange medical condition."

The next two days were a whirlwind as Brendan prepared for his lengthy stay in the hospital. Even though he was immersed in getting ready, he couldn't help but think about the time he was admitted to the Dungannon hospital with similar symptoms after passing out in French class two years earlier. When he told Professor Besser about his experience,

Professor Besser contacted the hospital for a full report. Professor Besser explained to him that not only had he been investigated for, but that he had also been diagnosed with pituitary gigantism. Professor Besser was astonished at the lack of urgency displayed and the fact that Brendan and his parents were not told about the potential dangers of gigantism. "I was extremely angry at the time, but as time passed my anger diminished, and I have become more philosophical about the poor health care I received." While the two-year delay worsened his condition, he found solace knowing that he was in a world-class endocrinology department receiving excellent care.

After Brendan was admitted to the hospital and started undergoing the testing needed to figure out his treatment plan, he became increasingly distressed about the surgery he might have to undergo. "The standard treatment at that time was surgical removal of the tumor, a particularly intrusive process involving an incision from the forehead over the skull to the back of the right ear. I was very, very scared of that option. I could see patients returning from surgery with their heads swathed in bandages. It was terrifying."

Relief flooded over him when Professor Besser told him that rather than the highly invasive surgery Brendan feared, the team found that radiotherapy was his best option. Each day for 25 days, Brendan received doses of radiation directed at the pituitary tumor. Brendan tolerated the treatment well with only a dull headache, a far cry from the violent headaches he long endured. He also received a series of hormone injections. They soon knew that the treatment was a success. "Within weeks of the treatment my growth hormone output plummeted, and much to my relief and joy, my delayed puberty set in. The treatment was more successful than I or even Professor Besser's team hoped."

After his release from the hospital, Brendan took a few weeks off to stay at his childhood home in Ackinduff "under the caring and watchful eye of my mother and regain my strength and vigor" before heading back to London to work. Despite the respite, when he returned to London, he began to develop troubling symptoms—breathlessness, coughing, fatigue, and a skin infection. He was taken by ambulance to St. Bartholomew's Hospital and placed in isolation. His diagnosis was pulmonary tuberculosis. Brendan was distraught but resolved. "How could this have happened to me after just recovering from my previous illness? I began to have doubts as whether I would ever reach old age, but I put them to the back of my mind and concentrated on getting well again."

Newly developed drugs to combat his tuberculosis gave Brendan hope, but the 13-week treatment plan tested his resolve. Unflagged, Brendan was determined to recover and build a new life for himself after his prolonged battle with his pituitary tumor and the subsequent challenge of getting tuberculosis. It was a long journey. Over the 15-month period since his first admission to St. Bartholomew's Hospital related to his pituitary tumor and his discharge after his second admission for tuberculosis, he spent six of the last 15 months in the hospital. His concerned parents encouraged him to return to Ackinduff where they could help him recover so that he could move on with his life. Brendan decided it was time to leave London behind and head back to his Irish homeland.

As he finished his diagnosis and treatment story, I felt deeply grateful that I met him and now knew another person who understood what it was like to have a body that did not go through normal growth and development. He understood what it was like to have blistering headaches, aching joints, and unresolved pain. He experienced the side-eyed glances and the unkind comments. He knew the difficulty of going through intense diagnostic testing, the relief of finally getting a diagnosis, and the fear of what the treatment plan would be.

# CHAPTER 3

# A HUMAN CURIOSITY: CHARLES BYRNE (1761-1783)

hen I first emailed Professor Korbonits in January 2021 to confirm I had the same *AIP* mutation found in her research, she not only sent me contact information for Brendan she also sent a YouTube link to the documentary *Charles Byrne: the Irish Giant/an Fathach Éireannach*[1] by Belfast filmmaker Ronan McCloskey in which Brendan played a prominent role. She told me that it also would help me to understand the link between Byrne, Brendan, me, and others with the Northern Ireland version of the *AIP* gene mutation, and it would give me insight into her research.

I read the dry biographical details of Charles Byrne's life in her research paper and knew that because we share the same *AIP* gene mutation, we are distant cousins. Nothing in the research paper prepared me for the heartbreaking details of Byrne's life captured in the documentary. I clicked on the YouTube link from Professor Korbonits and hit start.

The film opens in the Hunterian Museum at the Royal College of Surgeons in London. The focus is on the spotlighted skeleton of Charles Byrne standing in a glass display case. His bones are discolored brown, held together with wires, plates, and screws, a technique used by Dr. John Hunter, the man who put Byrne on display in 1783 as the centerpiece of

---

1 *Charles Byrne: the Irish Giant/an Fathach Éireannach*, directed by Ronan McCloskey (BBC Northern Ireland, 2011), https://www.youtube.com/watch?v=xLA-KZ7sBLg.

his collection of medical curiosities. The Irish language narration is sub-titled in English. I read along as I listen to the Irish intoned in the back-ground: This is the skeleton of Charles Byrne, the Irish Giant.

Next, the camera zooms in on Byrne's hand. I hit stop as a knot forms in my stomach. I flash back to 1976 and the very first medical test I had related to the diagnosis of my pituitary tumor: x-rays of my hands which showed the bony spade-like ends of my fingertips, a mark of acromegaly and gigantism. I peer closely at his hands and scrutinize the tips of his fingers. I see the spade-like ends that match mine. I see myself in Byrne.

I was captivated. I had to know more about Charles Byrne. When I first saw the documentary, I was shocked by the macabre tale of the short life of Charles Byrne who died when he was only 22 years old. I was equally fas-cinated by his story and yearned to know more about his life beyond what was covered in the film. Living in rural Virginia, especially during a pan-demic, made finding books or articles about an 18th century giant housed in a London museum difficult. Once again, my computer's search engine proved to be invaluable, when it led me to the digital library known as the Internet Archive (archive.org). The Archive unlocked Byrne's story through scanned 18th century newspaper articles, archived images of drawings from the 1780s, and advertisements for exhibits of giants at fairs and freak shows in England and Scotland. Over the next few months, I read everything I could find out about him. This is the story of my cousin Charles Byrne.

Born in 1761, Charles Byrne spent his early days in the lush farmlands and forests of Littlebridge, a village to the east of Cookstown on the border of Counties Tyrone and Derry, only a few miles from Brendan's home. Although it is uncertain exactly what his life was like in Ireland, his father was probably a linen weaver, his family quite poor, and his language Irish—all common demographics for Catholic peasants at the time.

Unlike his parents of average height, from an early age, Charles towered over the other children, and soon the adults, in the village. Villagers certainly thought of the Irish giants of legend like Fionn Mac Cumhaill and their supernatural powers when they saw him. He quickly learned that wherever he went, he was the center of attention.

News spread about his great height and people flocked to see him, curious to see someone of such exceptional stature. By 1780, Byrne was a local celebrity and joined the Tyrone military volunteers at Stewartstown where he served as the head of the recruitment parades despite being only 19 years old. He continued to draw large crowds to his local community, but he wanted more than local acclaim. As I read about life in Ireland at the time, it was clear to me why he was eager to leave behind the back-breaking work of raising flax and weaving it into linen. The physical labor would have been doubly challenging for him, given how gigantism most likely impacted his body with joint pain and headaches with no medical relief to ease his pain. He wanted a better life, and his remarkable height was his ticket to success.

Demand was high for giants willing to exhibit themselves in London and Edinburgh. A local villager Joe Vance seized the opportunity to use Charles to escape the rural life as well and convinced Charles to sign on with him as his manager and head to the British Isles to make money. Charles agreed and left his Irish world behind. They set off for Edinburgh in 1781, with plans to work their way south to London. Billed as an 8 feet 2 inches (249 cm) tall Irish Giant, Byrne quickly found welcoming audiences in Scotland at local fairs and festivals where spectators marveled at his great stature. Thrilled audiences gazed up in wonder at Charles who loomed over them. His time in Edinburgh burnished his reputation, especially when a local nightwatchman reported how Byrne lit his pipe using a streetlamp.[2]

---

2 John Kobler, *The Reluctant Surgeon: A Biography of John Hunter* (Akadine Press, 1999), 238.

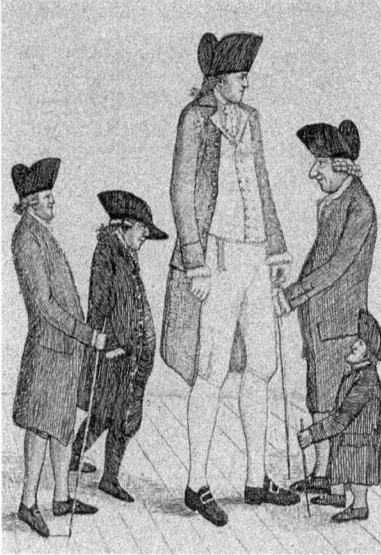

Charles Byrne with Scottish notables

As news of his amazing height spread, the duo continued through Northern England and on to London in search of larger audiences and greater pay. Ever ready to capitalize on Byrne's fame, Vance set Byrne up in a permanent viewing room so that he could charge spectators admission for the privilege of seeing Byrne every day instead of the few days of exhibiting time that a festival afforded. Competition in London was fierce. There was a robust market for the newest, rarest, tallest, or most unusual looking giant. Byrne fit the bill.

When Byrne arrived in London on April 11, 1782, he was already a celebrity. Vance took out an advertisement in *The Morning Herald* on April 24 to proclaim the Irish Giant's arrival.

> IRISH GIANT. To be seen this, and every day this week, in his large elegant room, at the cane shop, next door to late Cox's Museum, Spring Gardens, Mr. Byrne, the surprising Irish Giant, who is allowed to be the tallest man in the world; his height is eight feet two inches, and in full proportion accordingly; only 21 years of age. His stay will not be long in London, as he proposes shortly to visit the Continent.

At the time, London was a cosmopolitan city of nearly one million people dominated by opportunities for international commerce, trade, fashion, and ideas. It was also a city of despair with intense poverty, open sewers, ragged beggars, and rampant street-level crime—a magnet for all classes and occupations. Scientists and cutpurses, prostitutes and shop-keepers, tradesmen and gentry all crowded onto its bustling throughfares drawn by the city's culture, power, and diversions like the Bartholomew Fair. Byrne decided that the Bartholomew Fair, limited to just a few days in September, was the perfect place to attract attention and advertise his on-going appearance in his viewing room after the fair was over.

An 18th-century barrage of sights, smells, and sounds greeted raucous visitors to the annual Bartholomew Fair. A spectacle for the entirety of London whether upper or lower class, the fair drew merrymakers who crowded on to the fairgrounds in the Smithfield area near St. Bartholomew's Hospital to drink, gawk, and revel at the alcohol-fueled festival.

Capering clowns in flamboyant colors dazzled, conjurors wove their magic, and smoky sausages sizzled on braziers as hurdy-gurdy music jangled and the stench of dung wafted over the crowd from the nearby Smithfield stockyards. Hawkers beckoned visitors to part with a few pence to stare at the wonders of contortionists, acrobats, and wrestlers or gape at a two-headed cow, a six-legged ram, or a "learned" pig[3] who could tell someone's fortune with a tap of its snout to the tarot cards arrayed in front of it.

Physical disability as spectacle was on full display. An armless man thumped a drum with his feet. A woman with stunted limbs wailed a pathetic tune. The morbidly obese, dwarves, and natives from exotic lands proved popular as the spectators paused to take in the carnival antics, strange animals, and unusual humans. The sensational, the mysterious, and the grotesque titillated and amused.[4]

The extremes of the human body got the most interest and commanded the highest prices, but none proved more popular than the giants. Competing among the jostling urban whirlwind of gaudy colors, exotic showmanship,

---

3 Richard D. Altick, *The Shows of London* (Harvard University Press, 1978), 40.

4 Henry Morley, *Memoirs of Bartholomew Fairs* (originally published in 1857; George Routledge and Sons, London, 1892), 246-247.

and garish displays, a steady stream of giants, including Byrne, exhibited themselves over the 700 years of Bartholomew Fair history, from 1133 to 1855. Despite having been to Edinburgh, Scotland, Byrne must have been amazed at the spectacle of London's Bartholomew Fair, and I can imagine that fairgoers were equally astounded by Byrne's great height.

For Irish Giant Charles Byrne, the city promised prominence and prosperity as he strode down the streets of London in 1782 to his lodgings in Charing Cross after the fair. He had no way of knowing that a pituitary tumor caused his great height, but he was ready to take full advantage of his stature to make money.

Byrne took the London entertainment world by storm. "Elegantly dressed in a frock coat, waistcoat, knee breeches, silk stockings, frilled cuffs and collar, topped by a three-cornered hat, Byrne spoke graciously with his thunderous voice and displayed the refined manners of a gentleman."[5] In his viewing room in Charing Cross, he commanded top dollar, charging two shillings sixpence per person,[6] with eager spectators lining up from 11:00 am to 3:00 pm and from 5:00 pm to 8:00 pm six days a week. Newspaper accounts shortly after his arrival describe him as a "modern living Colossus" and "a prodigy," with "elegance, symmetry, and proportion of this wonderful phenomenon in nature."[7] Byrne was in his prime as an entertainer.

I was impressed by who met Byrne in the early days of his time in London. By August 12, 1782, Byrne had met King George III, the Duke and Duchess of Devonshire, and Lady Spencer. He made his mark with the Royal Society national scientific academy when they speculated on the cause of his extraordinary height.

---

5 Eric Cubbage, "The Tragic Story of Charles Byrne 'The Irish Giant,'" web.archive.org/web/20111008234246/http://www.thetallestman.com/pdf/charlesbyrne.pdf.

6 Approximately £28.77 or $36.44 in 2023.

7 *The Morning Herald*, 6 May 1782.

In perhaps the greatest acknowledgement of the young giant's popularity, London-based Theatre Royal in the Haymarket opened a new summer play, "Harlequin Teague: or the Giant's Causeway," which boasted packed houses throughout August. Much to my delight, I was able to find a detailed description and review of the play in the 1782 *Town and Country Magazine* in the Internet Archive, which showed the parallel between Byrne and the play's lead character Teague.

The traditional pantomime play begins at the Giant's Causeway in Ireland during a raging storm. Entrapped in a rock by an evil spirit, Cormac, the leader of the giants, escapes his prison when lightning strikes the rock during the tempest. He sees the lead character Teague and demands to know why fellow giant Teague is standing there. Teague replies that "being very poor, he has a vast inclination to become rich and hearing that London was the only place where a man stood a chance of gaining abundance from doing nothing, he was making the best of his way hither." Cormac presents Teague with a sword and changes him into Harlequin, a stock character from the commedia dell'arte theatre known for his comic timing and slapstick antics. Mirroring Byrne's journey from Ireland, Teague sets off sword in hand to seize his fortune in London.[8]

In only five months, Byrne's celebrity status in London as the tallest and most unusual giant seemed assured. However, the whirlwind that brought him fame and fortune was threatening to become a maelstrom. The pituitary tumor that caused his system to be flooded with growth hormone gave him the gift of his famous height, but it also exacted its price.

For Byrne, every day was a day filled with the pain of aching joints and splitting headaches. While alcohol may have lessened his pain—he was reputed to drink excessively—the relief was only temporary. As I read

---

8 *The Town and Country Magazine, Or, Universal Repository of Knowledge, Instruction, and Entertainment*: Volume 14, August 1782, 400.

about his life, it broke my heart to think about how young he was when he first came to London. He was only 21 years old.

His life by this point had to be one of pain and constant pressure to perform for the spectators that came to stare at him. To add to his difficulties, he also caught the eye of one of London's leading scientists, a man known for his surgical skills and deep curiosity about human anatomy. He is now considered to be the father of modern surgery, but in Byrne's day he was a man obsessed with searching for and collecting specimens for his museum of medical curiosities and human oddities.

That man was Dr. John Hunter.

Hunter was born on February 14, 1728, the youngest of ten children in a farming family. From an early age, John loved to wander the hillsides of Lanarkshire, Scotland. Unlike his studious older brother, William, who at an early age was sent off to Glasgow to become a doctor, John detested school and "skipped lessons to go rambling through the woods and fields, stalking wild animals in the undergrowth."[9] His hatred of books was legendary.

By the time John was 13 years old, he abandoned school while his brother William, ten years his senior, thrived as a doctor. By the time William was thirty, he moved to England to build his physician practice by delivering babies for London's upper class.[10] William tempered his Scottish upbringing, navigated Georgian society, and established himself as a doctor to the elite.

Using his expertise and connections, William created an anatomy school to attract aspiring surgeons eager to learn dissection. The school

9 Wendy Moore, *The Knife Man: Blood, Body Snatching, and the Birth of Modern Surgery* (New York: Broadway Books, 2005), 16.

10 Ibid., 13.

was an unexpected success, and William knew it was time to hire an assistant. Although he had not seen John in many years and he was unsure if his awkward, uncultured, and largely uneducated country brother[11] could transition to life in London, William invited John to be his assistant in 1748. When John arrived, he quickly learned dissection and put his new skills to the test as an anatomist.

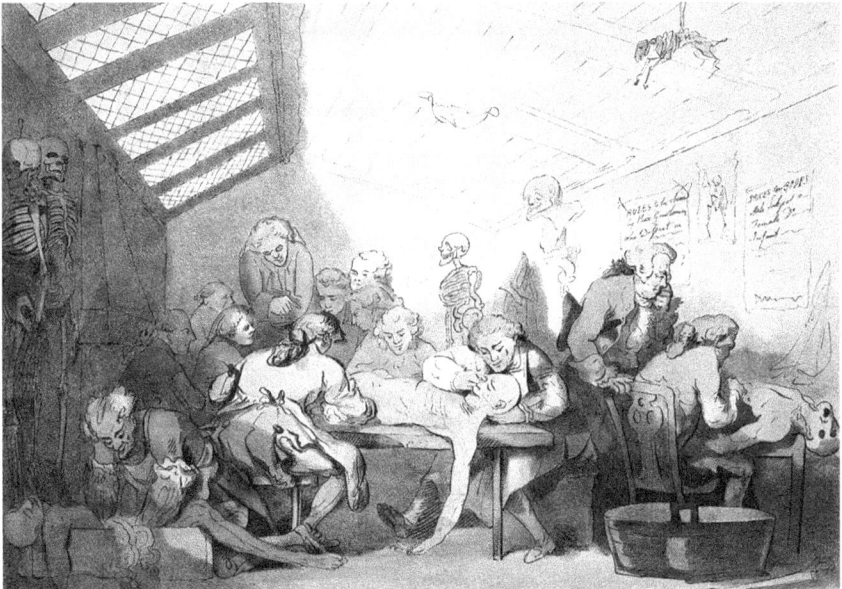

*The Dissecting Room* by Rowlandson with John Hunter to the far right.

A bone saw clanked as it hit the side of the metal basin to John's right side while another vessel caught bodily fluids dripping off the cold plank where the cadaver sprawled. John, scalpel in hand, stared at the corpse in front of him. The stink of rotting corpses and putrid viscera permeated the air in his brother William's dissection room located in the rear of his home on Great Windmill Street in London. The dead body was one of

11 Ibid., 14.

more than 2000 cadavers that John Hunter dissected over the 12 years he spent as his brother's pupil and assistant.

Determination to understand the human body, a strong stomach to endure the stench, and the agility to cut apart a corpse rapidly before the body decomposed in the days before formaldehyde was used as an embalming agent were all vital skills of an anatomist. John had them all. Providing the steady supply of dead bodies needed for the study of anatomy—a key part of his apprenticeship with his brother—was a skill he needed to learn.

At first, John relied on workhouses or prisons for the cadavers, which offered up a few of their unclaimed poor or executed prisoners as subjects for the anatomists. However, as other anatomy schools formed in London, demand for those corpses outstripped the supply. John responded by organizing the anatomy students into nighttime raids, creeping into graveyards to find bodies. Soon, even that tactic didn't provide the number of corpses needed, given the small window of opportunity for dissection due to the rapid decay of the prized corpses. The need for cadavers at his brother's growing anatomy school demanded a more efficient solution, so John turned next to the resurrectionists.[12]

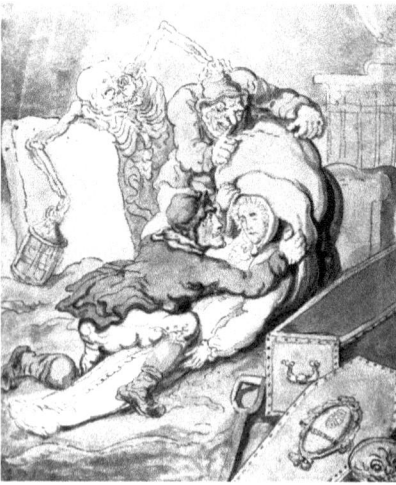

Two resurrectionists snatch a corpse while Death looks on

Professional body-snatchers, also known as resurrectionists or sack-'em-up men, exhumed dead bodies for a price, with unusual, malformed, or difficult-to-obtain corpses bringing a premium. No one was safe from

12 James Moores Ball, *The Body Snatchers* (New York: Dorset Press, 1928), 68-70.

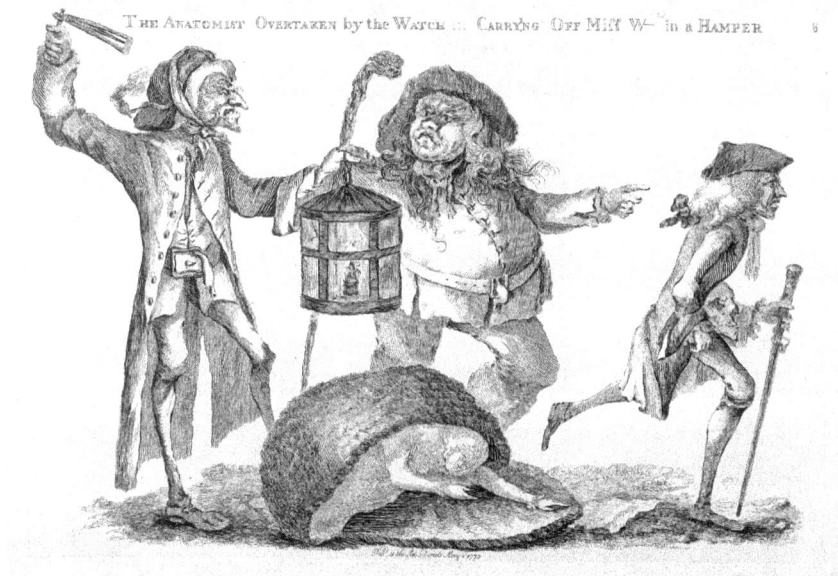

THE ANATOMIST OVERTAKEN by the WATCH ... CARRYING OFF MISS W— in a HAMPER

Two watchmen catch an anatomist stealing a corpse

their clutches. Women who died in late pregnancy from eclampsia were prized for the obstetrical secrets their fetuses provided. A child, known as a small, brought a lesser price than an adult corpse unless a birth defect was found which led to a negotiated price based on the deformity. Paupers in an open mass grave provided the resurrectionists with a bonanza of dead bodies, but the pit drew other nocturnal predators. Mangled bodies barely fetched enough money to warrant the risk of grave robbing.

Technically in the 1780s, stealing a dead body, unlike the clothes found on the body, was not a crime, so the legal risk was low. If the perpetrators took only the body and left the clothes, they may have violated societal norms, but they were not considered to be robbers. London society was horrified at the thought of dissection, a fate associated with criminals, and relatives took great pains to protect gravesites from the body snatchers. The resurrectionists became increasingly cunning and efficient. They posed as family members to take away the corpse before it was buried.

They worked skillfully and swiftly in teams with a system to dig down to the coffin, break through the lid, lift out the corpse, strip the body, place it in a sack, re-seal the coffin, and return the dirt to the gravesite. Thirty minutes later, the sack-'em-up men were gone. The grave looked untouched.

After twelve years at his brother's anatomy school, John Hunter moved on to develop his own career in medicine and no longer had to get cadavers for his brother. However, he continued to be an anatomist for his entire life, which demanded that he continue his search for bodies to dissect. The resurrectionists knew that Hunter paid the highest prices for unusual specimens, and when Hunter created his own dissection room at the back of his house, a rap on the door meant there was a fresh specimen to dissect if only he paid their rate. His lifetime collection of dissected specimens for his museum continued to grow.

By 1782, Hunter amassed more than 14,000 specimens, both animal and human, which he planned to display in a museum at the home he was building at 28 Leicester Square in London. As the workmen put the finishing touches on Hunter's gallery of medical curiosities which he hoped to open in 1783, Hunter began to envision a centerpiece for his exhibition. He did not have to look far for a magnificent specimen. As a Londoner, Hunter knew that the Irish giant Charles Byrne was a sensation. While Hunter knew about gigantism and the trajectory of the illness—information that might have helped Byrne—he was more interested in obtaining Byrne's body after death than helping him to cope with his disease during his life. Although Hunter didn't know the exact cause of gigantism, he knew the course of Byrne's disease: Byrne would most likely die quite young. Realizing Byrne was 21 years old, Hunter knew that he had found his centerpiece. He only needed to wait for him to die and be willing to pay the price.

Just as Hunter set his sights on Byrne in November 1782, Byrne's fortune began to falter. While Byrne had taken London by storm only seven months prior, the public's desire for the latest, greatest, tallest, or most unusual made it difficult to maintain his celebrity status. The crowds started to dwindle. To save money, his manager Joe Vance moved Byrne from Charing Cross to a cheaper lodging at Piccadilly, in the hopes of continuing to cash in on Byrne. While keeping admission of two shillings for ladies and gentlemen, he lowered admission for children and servants to one shilling in hopes of drawing in the working-class residents of Piccadilly.

By early 1783, the spectators that once crowded into Byrne's residence slowed to a trickle, just as competition heated up from other giants eager to profit from the public's intense interest in sideshows by setting themselves up as exhibits.[13] Making their debut as the Gigantic Irish Twins after growing up in the same village as Byrne, the 7 foot 2 inches tall (218 cm) Knipe brothers arrived in London from the north of Ireland. They knocked Byrne out of the limelight, giving spectators the thrill of seeing the identical twin giants for the price of one. Further displacing Byrne in the public's eye, Patrick Cotter, known as the Bristol Giant or the Irish Giant, arrived on the scene. He adopted the name Patrick O'Brien as his stage name to emphasize his Irish heritage and to bolster his claim that he was a direct descendent of King Brian Boru, the legendary giant and Irish hero who defeated all attackers to become the High King of Ireland in 1002 A.D. Cotter deliberately set himself up as a rival to Byrne through advertisements that claimed he was more than four inches taller than Byrne.[14]

By the end of March 1783, only a year after his arrival in London, Byrne's world began to unravel. The damage from the pituitary tumor was reaching its peak. He was dogged by splitting headaches, throbbing joints, and crippling pain. Alcohol dampened the pain, but his excessive

---

13 Wouter W. de Herder, "Acromegalic Gigantism, Physicians and Body Snatching: Past or Present?," *Pituitary* 15, no. 3 (2012): 312.

14 Graham Frankcom and Jonathan H. Musgrave, *The Irish Giant* (London: Gerald Duckworth & Co., 1976), 22.

drinking only added to his woes. Always a fan of the local taverns, Byrne began to drink more heavily, appearing disheveled, and slumping in a chair at his exhibitions.

Byrne once again moved to cheaper quarters—this time on Cockspur Street—and lowered admission to a mere one shilling for all spectators. To make matters worse, his unscrupulous manager Joe Vance deserted him, leaving Byrne alone in London, his prospects dim. His hope of continued fame extinguished.

Despite his descent, Byrne managed to save more than £700, a sum worth more than £137,000 today. However, misfortune haunted Byrne. *The Morning Herald* newspaper, dated April 23, 1783, reported Byrne's fate.

> The Irish Giant, a few evenings since, taking a lunar ramble, was tempted to visit the Black Horse, a little public-house facing the King's mews; and before he returned to his own apartments, found himself a less man than he had been the beginning of the evening, by the loss of upwards of 700£ in bank notes, which had been taken out of his pocket.

With nearly all his money stolen, abandoned, in pain, and alone, Charles Byrne was a shattered man. He came to London to find fame and fortune. He found both, only to lose everything.

Meanwhile, John Hunter, eager to add Byrne to his collection, watched Byrne's descent with rapt interest. Using his connections as an anatomist, Hunter notified the resurrectionists that he would pay a premium for the giant's body upon delivery. He hired spies to keep watch over Byrne's deteriorating condition. He even went as far as to hire one of the body-snatchers named Howieson to move into an apartment on Cockspur Street near Byrne's lodgings. He told Howieson to report back to him at once when Byrne died. When Hunter learned about the robbery, he saw his chance to guarantee that Byrne would be his. He offered Byrne £50 for his body.

Appalled, Byrne refused. Not only was Byrne repulsed by the idea of being dissected like a common criminal, but he also feared that his mutilated body would be unfit for the Last Judgement Day when his body came back to join with his spirit. He turned to some fellow Irishmen he knew to save him from the anatomist's knife. Byrne begged them to bury him at sea far from the clutches of the body-snatchers and the cold plank in Hunter's dissection room. They promised to protect him, and with his last few pounds, Byrne pre-paid the undertaker to carry out his wishes.

While Hunter may have been the most blatant about his obsession with obtaining Byrne's body, he was not the only anatomist in London who wanted to dissect Byrne to learn the secrets of his great height. To thwart competition from other surgeons and outwit Byrne, Hunter continued to pay Howieson to watch Byrne's every move and report back on his worsening condition. Hunter did not have long to wait.[15]

On Sunday, June 1, 1783, Charles Byrne died at the age of 22 in his Cockspur Street lodging. Local newspapers announced his death:

> Charles Byrne, the famous Irish giant, whose death is said to have been precipitated by excessive drinking, to which he was always addicted, but more particularly since his late loss of almost all of his property, which he had simply invested in a single bank note of £700. In his last moments (it has been said) that he requested that his ponderous remains might be thrown into the sea, in order that his bones might be placed far out of the reach of the chirurgical fraternity.[16]

London's surgeons demanded Byrne's body be given up for dissection. Competition was fierce as reported by *The Morning Herald* on June 5, 1783.

---

15 John Kobler, *The Reluctant Surgeon: A Biography of John Hunter* (New York: Akadine Press, 1999), 240.

16 *Gentleman's Magazine*, 53 (1783): 541.

The whole tribe of surgeons put in a claim for the poor
departed Irish Giant, and surrounded his house just as
Greenland harpooners would an enormous whale. One of
them has gone so far as to have a niche made for himself in
the giant's coffin, in order to his being ready at hand, on the
"witching time of night, when church-yards yawn.

Despite the demands, Byrne's Irish protectors stuck with their agreement. They stood guard to prevent the theft of Byrne's body. However,
after they placed him in an enormous coffin, they couldn't resist trying
to make money from Byrne. Hoping to profit from Byrne's demise, they
charged two shillings sixpence to see his massive casket. Finally, on June
6, the undertaker loaded the coffin onto the funeral wagon for transport
to Margate by the sea seventy-five miles away. After chartering a boat, the
Irishmen believed that they fulfilled Byrne's final wishes as they watched
the enormous coffin slip beneath the waters of the North Sea.

Sadly, Byrne's story does not end there. In a chilling twist, his coffin
may have been laid to rest in the sea's watery depths, but Byrne's body
was not inside. No one knows for sure how his body was stolen. Only
John Hunter knows the truth of how he was able to secure Byrne's corpse
by fooling Byrne's fellow Irishmen into thinking that they buried him at
sea. John Kobler in his book *The Reluctant Surgeon* offers one version of
what happened:

When Byrne finally died, the watchers, stripped the corpse, so
that if caught, they could not be charged with stealing property. They nailed shut the empty casket and lugged the body
down the stairs. John was waiting in his coach, and Howieson
was perched on the driver seat. Money and corpse swiftly
changed hands. Then clattering through the stilled streets,
the coach sped straight on under the lightning sky to Earl's

Court, the tense little surgeon, and the huge naked cadaver jouncing together in the cramped blackness of the rear seat.[17]

Another popular theory blames the undertaker in a story that emphasizes the lengths Hunter would go to obtain the body. After Howieson notified Hunter of Byrne's death, Hunter quickly found the undertaker and bribed him with the exorbitant sum of £500 (more than £85,000 in 2023) to switch Byrne's body for stones in the casket. Hunter then loaded up the body and scurried off to his dissection room. Either story could be true or neither one. None of the stories have been verified. What is certain though is that Hunter obtained the body.

The story then takes another bizarre twist—a turn that is hard to understand given Hunter's obsession with obtaining Byrne's body for dissection to learn its secrets. Rather than putting Byrne under the scalpel, Hunter dismembered the body and boiled it to de-flesh the bones. Perhaps he was fearful of retribution from the Irishmen tricked into believing that Byrne's corpse was at the bottom of the sea or worried that other surgeons would condemn him for hoarding the corpse for himself. The bones stayed a secret for four years as Hunter waited for interest in the Irish giant to abate. In 1787, after wiring Byrne's bones together, Hunter quietly put the skeleton, the centerpiece for his museum of curiosities at his home on Leicester Square, on display .

Six years later, in 1793, Hunter died suddenly while vigorously debating the merits of allowing two young Scots to enroll at St. George's Hospital despite their lack of a formal education, just as Hunter himself started as an apprentice. As requested, his body was taken to his dissection room at his Leicester Square home where he was autopsied and later buried. His son Clift kept his museum collection at Leicester Square until 1799 when the British Government purchased the massive collection of

---

17 John Kobler, *The Reluctant Surgeon: A Biography of John Hunter* (New York: Akadine Press, 1999), 243.

anatomical specimens, articulated skeletons, and surgical instruments for £15,000 (equivalent to £2.1 million in 2023). The government transferred custody of the collection to the Company of Surgeons (renamed the following year the Royal College of Surgeons) and moved the artifacts to the Royal College's new building at Lincoln's Inn Fields[18] where it was established as the Hunterian Museum. Frozen in time and suspended in a glass display case as the centerpiece in the Crystal Gallery, Charles Byrne's mortal remains served as a tribute to the very man who stalked him in life and profited from his death.

For me, meeting Charles Byrne through the documentary was a profound emotional experience, but it was a two-dimensional one. He was an image on my computer monitor, my view controlled by the camera's lens as it zoomed in on his hands and panned out to his full skeleton in its glass display case. On the other hand, Brendan's experience of meeting Byrne was very real, and I was able to see his reaction which was captured in the documentary.

The scene opens with the camera following Brendan and Professor Korbonits as they enter the Crystal Gallery in the Hunterian Museum. The camera focuses on Brendan as he walks past exhibits of Hunter's medical curiosities. In the film, I could see sealed glass apothecary jars holding excised tumors and distorted fetuses, their forms floating eerily in clear liquid. I could also see misshapen human skulls lining one shelf and wooden tablets with dry-mounted blood vessels resting on another as Brendan approached the towering 240-year-old skeleton of Charles Byrne. Brendan stands there; his eyes riveted on Byrne's skeleton. I could hear him catch his breath and then let out a deep sigh.

---

18 Wendy Moore, *The Knife Man: Blood, Body Snatching, and the Birth of Modern Surgery* (New York: Broadway Books, 2005), 268-269.

I asked him what he was thinking when he saw Byrne for the first time during the filming'. Brendan said that he couldn't help but reflect on his own journey. "I knew I was looking at his earthly remains, and that his spirit was elsewhere, but my imme- diate reaction was not one of shock, as I prepared myself as

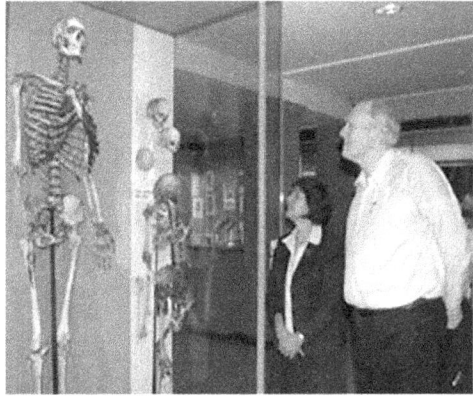

Charles Byrne, Professor Korbonits, and Brendan

to what I was about to see. I stared at him for a time, and I could only feel enormous sympathy for the man."

He went on to tell me about how he felt after Professor Korbonits pointed out some of the differences between a normal skeleton unaffected by excess growth hormone and Byrne's. "She told me that he was still growing when he died as his long bones in his legs and arms had not fused. I remember thinking that here in the starkest terms was a representation of me when I was diagnosed in 1972. This is how I may have ended up without treatment." Despite the centuries between their lives, Brendan felt that he knew what it was like to be Charles Byrne. "His struggle with his advanced condition in the last years of his life must have been a miser- able existence." Brendan also reflected on how difficult it must have been for Byrne to have any kind of normal life because of his stature.

Brendan and I have talked about how we both were keenly aware of how different we looked from others around us before we were treated for our tumors. We both have stories of being stared at or feeling side-eyed glances when someone was not bold enough to gawk.

Brendan told me a story of how he remembers seeing people react when they saw him. The reactions varied from staring open-mouthed to nudging the person next to them and saying loudly, "God, would you look at that man." He told me about a time when as a teenager "a silly woman asked me to get out of my car so that her children could see me. I explained that I was not a circus act. She was most displeased." Brendan noted that Byrne was even more striking because he was an extra foot taller than Brendan in a time when people in general were much shorter than they are now. "It must have been a very unhappy existence with gawping people lining up to see him."

Brendan and I have also spoken many times about how grateful we are to Charles Byrne. Major contributions to the understanding of gigantism and acromegaly are a direct result of scientific research conducted on Byrne's skeleton. We are the beneficiaries of that research. However, we are appalled by how Dr. Hunter's insatiable curiosity and desire to have Byrne as a prize specimen for his vast collection denied Byrne his wish to be buried at sea. The social values of 18th-century London that allowed Hunter to stalk Byrne while he was living and buy his corpse when he died are hard to accept with our 21st-century minds.

For more than 200 years, the skeletal remains of Charles Byrne hung in the Hunterian Museum to be stared at. He was a captivating object—a gruesome relic in a glass box with a macabre backstory of body-snatchers and a fixated physician from the 1700s. In May 2017, the museum closed for renovations, and Charles Byrne's skeleton was removed and placed in storage. The closure of the Hunterian Museum for renovations reignited a longstanding controversy surrounding the repatriation of Charles Byrne's skeleton. Advocates for Byrne's repatriation argued that his remains should be buried at sea as he wanted. Opponents of repatriation cited the scientific and historical value of Byrne's remains, highlighting the insights they offered into medical history and human anatomy. They argued that his skeleton should remain accessible for research and education purposes. In 2023, the museum decided to discontinue the skeleton's public display but allow the skeleton to remain in the collection to be used for scientific research.

# CHAPTER 4

# FOCUSING THE LENS

When I look back on the days after I met Brendan in January 2021, I am reminded of how restricted my life was during the pandemic. It was a time of constantly calculating risk and assessing the safety of even the most mundane activities, such as grocery shopping. Our library was closed. The in-person 5K races that I loved as an avid runner shifted to virtual ones and even those were few and far between. The news was dismal as doctors and nurses struggled to keep up with the rising death toll. The pandemic raged, but there was hope when I was able to get the Covid vaccine in March 2021. Maybe one day I could fly to Ireland to meet Brendan and see the land of my ancestors.

In the meantime, collaborating with Brendan on a book about our experiences with gigantism was a welcome break from the pandemic. My real life may have been confined, but my online world expanded when Brendan connected me with Ronan, the director of the documentary, so that I could understand his role in Brendan's life and Professor Korbonits' research.

Brendan told me about Ronan's affinity for off-beat topics in Irish culture—his films include Irish sumo wrestlers, Irish robot camel racers, and paranormal Irish pet communicators—which opened him to exploring unusual avenues in Irish history. His passion for the Irish language matched well with funding from Northern Ireland Screen's Irish Language Broadcast Fund to film the documentary in Irish, Byrne's language, with English subtitles. His love of Irish legends and mythology helped him draw parallels between Byrne's story and the stories he remembered from his time growing up in Omagh so close to the geographic hotspot for gigantism. It was clear that he was an ideal choice to direct and produce the film.

When I watched the documentary, I was struck by how well Ronan was able to intertwine Byrne's 18th-century history with Brendan's modern-day discovery of his own gigantism while explaining details of Professor Korbonits' research. He used a combination of actors recreating scenes from Byrne's life, documentary footage of Brendan and Professor Korbonits, and filmed interviews with Brendan's brother Aiden and cousin Niamh to tie all three elements of the documentary together. I was fascinated by Ronan's technical abilities as a director and curious to know how he persuaded Brendan and Professor Korbonits to take part in the documentary. Brendan continued to keep in touch with Ronan after the filming of the documentary, so he sent me Ronan's email address.

I emailed Ronan, and he replied with a Zoom invitation, which I gladly accepted. It turned out that he was just as interested in meeting me as I was in him, given that Brendan told him that I was the first person in the United States identified with the Northern Irish variant of the *AIP* genetic mutation.

When he popped up on my screen for the Zoom meeting, I was won over at once by his lively nature and enthusiasm. I was intrigued by the whiteboard that I could see over his shoulder which was covered with scribbles in black marker and plastered with sticky notes that showed the details of his current film project. I could almost see the workings of his creative mind displayed through the connections mapped out on the whiteboard. It was easy to jump right into a conversation with him about the genesis and development of the documentary.

Ronan told me that in 2009 BBC Northern Ireland decided to commission a documentary about Byrne and hired Ronan as the director/producer. The original plan for the documentary was a straightforward biography, focusing on Byrne as an Irish giant and symbol of strength.

Although Ronan grew up in Omagh only 25 miles from Byrne's home near Cookstown, he had never heard of Byrne. "Surprisingly, I'd never heard anything about him. For whatever reason, very few people had. I don't even think the editor heard of him before there was talk of making a film about him. Byrne definitely wasn't something that was in the imagination of Northern Irish people."

Although he hadn't heard of Byrne, Ronan remembered other stories about giants in Omagh. "I remember hearing about an old man in the area named Peadar who said that a giant had lain down in the forest and that somebody cut his outline round with a spade. There his outline remained until that small wood was cut down in the Second World War." Ronan told me that he believed that the story was part of the oral history of where he lived, which in time became solidified into local mythology and folklore. "A story like this has a kind of supernatural feel to it. It shows that the giant had power."

Despite knowing nothing about Byrne, Ronan accepted the commission and traveled to London to continue his research for the documentary. His first stop was the Hunterian Museum. When he saw Byrne's skeleton, Ronan was amazed by his size and thought back to the story he came across about Byrne leading a parade through Stewartstown. "I know others saw him as just another big strong Irish man, but I think there's another reason. He was at the front of that parade because he was just an incredible medical case." Ronan told me just how astonishing it was to see Byrne and how impressed he was by Byrne's sheer physical presence "Until you actually see him, you don't really understand what it must have been like for people then to see him."

While there, Ronan met with the museum curator to learn more about Byrne's life and history. By chance, the curator told him about Professor Korbonits' research into the genetics of gigantism. This fortuitous remark took his documentary far beyond the simple biography of Byrne that was originally envisioned. A phone call to Professor Korbonits was the obvious next step. It was only after talking with Professor Korbonits that he learned about the medical condition that caused Byrne's height. "I realized the documentary had so much more of a story to tell because the story of Charles Byrne had never been fully told. It was always that he was a guy who went to London and became a drunken Irishman and then died. Whereas in reality, this guy had untreated gigantism in a very extreme form."

When Ronan contacted his editor to let him know about the medical researcher and her interest in testing Charles Byrne's skeleton to see if he had the same genetic mutation, it was clear to both that the documentary needed to shift its storyline to include Professor Korbonits' findings. "We realized that we had quite a story here. It was becoming a medical mystery story. Even my editor said, 'God, could Byrne have had the same genetic mutation 250 years ago?'" Ronan decided to contact Professor Korbonits again and ask her to meet him in London to be in the documentary. Professor Korbonits' analysis of the skeleton and her genetic research promised to be a vital part of Charles Byrne's story.

I asked Professor Korbonits why she was willing to connect with a filmmaker. Typically, art and science exist in separate realms, and opening the research process to outside scrutiny from a journalist or documentarian can be fraught. "Doctors don't usually talk to journalists but the reason that I met him was because he said that he came through the museum. I thought meeting this guy couldn't do any harm, so I met him, and he was very genuine. He looks right into your eyes. We built up a relationship, and I started to trust him. As it turned out, I was quite right to trust him."

Eventually, Professor Korbonits' confidence would be repaid as Ronan moved from being a chronicler of her research into being an active participant by helping her understand the area in Northern Ireland that through her research would come to be known as a geographic hotspot for gigantism.

Once he secured Professor Korbonits' cooperation for his documentary, Ronan turned his attention to his childhood home in Omagh to continue his research for the film. He recalled a time he overheard his father. "I remember being in our house and someone telling my father about a person they knew as a child who couldn't stop growing. They continued on about another child with the same problem. This was in 1982 or so. Funny, I even knew then it wasn't a good thing at all. My father was a dentist, so he understood it was a medical condition. I wonder if those children turned out to be giants now."

Ronan decided to travel through the geographic hotspot for the genetic mutation east of his parents' home to visit what is believed to be Charles Byrne's home in Littlebridge near Cookstown. "I met somebody just sitting at her house and when I told her I was there because I knew someone had lived there with gigantism, she immediately started to think. She said, to be sure there's a family up the road, two of them have that." Ronan continued to talk with others in the area, only to hear more tales of giants who had lived there.

Knowing that there was a possibility that modern-day giants might be living in the area, Ronan contacted a local historian to see if he had information about anyone with gigantism in the region. "He said to me, there's a man in Killeeshil and he's brave and tall. Brave is something we would say to mean he's very tall. So, I said, how tall is he? And he told me that he stood to the edge of the house but was able to bend over to come in. And I said, what is he called? He said, Brendan Holland."

Ronan tried at once to find Brendan through a Google search. He was able to find to obtain his contact information through the local historical society. He emailed Brendan, telling him that he was doing a project on the history of County Tyrone and pituitary gigantism. "Brendan phoned me up, and he said I can help you on both counts. So, I drove up to see him and as soon as I saw him, I thought, you're booked. I knew that if I got him in it, the film would take off." Ronan now had a spokesperson for the patients with the disease of gigantism and an interesting angle for the documentary.

When Ronan met Brendan in his office in Dungannon, he filled Brendan in on the details of Byrne's life, his celebrity status in the 1780s, his early death at age 22, and the underhanded methods Dr. John Hunter used to obtain his skeleton. It was the first time that Brendan heard about Byrne. "I was amazed to find out that he was born 20 miles northeast of where I live and that he spent most of his life in the area until he went to London to seek his fortune. I could see the parallels in our lives, and I was hooked on this man. I had to know more."

Ronan convinced Brendan that it was important for him to come to London for the filming of the documentary. Ronan was certain that Brendan could provide insight into Byrne's mindset when he went to London, especially given how closely their lives aligned. They were the same age and were from the same area before they left Ireland to live in London. Brendan realized that Byrne had lived in Spring Gardens off Trafalgar Square, only a few hundred yards from his workplace in 1972. "As I learned more about the similarities in our lives and what we suffered having the same pituitary condition, I began to feel a certain closeness to this man despite the difference in the times that we lived."

Ronan also told him about Professor Korbonits and her research. Ronan explained how he was in contact with a professor in St Bartholomew's Hospital who was an authority on gigantism and that she was doing important research on the illness. Brendan's interest intensified when he learned that she was at the same hospital where he was diagnosed and treated 37 years prior. Brendan knew that if he could meet Professor Korbonits, he might get the answer to the question that vexed him for years. "Why me?" "Why did I develop gigantism?"

When Brendan agreed to be in the documentary and go to London to meet Professor Korbonits, Ronan realized he had the pieces in place to make an exceptional film. "It was amazing how this project just came to me. I had no idea what it was all about at first. I was just pulled in."

He knew that he had stumbled onto something special that captured not only his imagination as a filmmaker but also told a fascinating story of Irish strength and resolve. Brendan proved to be a symbol of that strength in his role as a spokesperson for people with gigantism in the film. "Brendan was able to give it all a human face. When you were with him, he was physically amazing, and you could see people be blown away a bit. He's so amazing, this big friendly man, who really goes over emotionally with people."

By fusing the art of storytelling with the science of genetic gigantism, filmmaker Ronan became a spark that led to a fuller understanding of what it is like to live with a rare disease like gigantism. Because Professor Korbonits was open to the artistic process, the documentary extended beyond the story of one historic giant to include the stories of modern-day giants living today with the disease and who are beneficiaries of Professor Korbonits' research. In exploring a broader narrative, the film tells the story of human suffering. As Ronan commented, "There's a real gravity to the story of Charles Byrne. Part of the gravity is the way it makes you reflect on how we observe others. He is a metaphor for human suffering as spectacle. It's not just about his pituitary gigantism. It's about the human condition."

# CHAPTER 5

# A STUDY IN TIME

I remember the incredible sense of wonder that washed over me when I realized that I was related to Charles Byrne and Brendan. I was equally fascinated with Professor Korbonits and her research, and how her scientific findings tied their storylines together. I felt like I was in a time machine that whisked me back to 2010 to see first-hand how Professor Korbonits' research developed in real time, as she hammered out the details of her genetic gigantism research that resulted in her paper that I found online. The documentary showed me how her research was not just words on a page. It brought to life the drama behind scientific discovery and showed the challenges researchers like Professor Korbonits face.

Brendan told me that he admired her willingness to connect with her patients, and I could see that directly in the film. Although Brendan had talked with Professor Korbonits on the phone, it was the documentary that recorded their first physical meeting. The film shows Brendan as he enters St. Bartholomew's Hospital's (Barts) historic central courtyard, with shade trees and wooden benches surrounding an elegant Victorian-era fountain. Then, across the courtyard, he sees Professor Korbonits and her welcoming smile headed his way, her hand outstretched. Brendan told me that as they shook hands, the warmth and caring that he so distinctly remembered from his time at Barts when he was diagnosed so long ago came flooding back. "The way that she had an instant relationship with Ronan, it was very much like that for me with her. We just clicked."

The more I delved into Professor Korbonits' work, the more I wanted to know how she came across Charles Byrne. How did she first meet him? I was also struck by how coincidence and serendipity played a role in her research, just as a chance Google search one boring afternoon led me to her. The documentary had a wealth of information about her work, and I was also able to find online recorded lectures and podcasts where she discussed the history of her work on genetic gigantism and the breadth of scientific inquiry that led to her publications. She also joined Brendan and me on a few of our Zoom meetings. Not only was the research itself intriguing, but the story behind how she learned about Charles Byrne and the Northern Ireland version of the *AIP* genetic mutation was equally absorbing.

Professor Korbonits came from Hungary to Barts as an endocrinology doctor in the early 1990s. By 2003, she had established herself as a clinical academic researcher with a prestigious Medical Research Council Clinician Scientist fellowship and expertise in pituitary tumorigenesis and growth hormone. She was very interested in how the body regulated growth, and she studied a novel hormone called ghrelin, which is implicated in growth hormone and appetite regulation. But her interests were not simply academic. Even as she conducted cutting-edge research, she continued to care for patients in the endocrinology department at Barts, gaining valuable insight into a wide range of endocrine disorders, including acromegaly. She saw first-hand how endocrine disease affected her patients, both physically and mentally.

Over time, she noticed that some of her patients with acromegaly had family members who also had the disease, an indicator that the disease might be genetic. "Barts had a seemingly high number of acromegaly patients coming to the hospital from Malta,[1] the island in the Mediterranean." Professor Besser, head of the endocrinology department and the appointed endocrinologist to the Maltese Government, thought something genetic must be going on to have so many acromegaly patients given the small population of Malta. Shortly after hearing his theory, she was at a conference in Europe, and luckily mentioned the observations to a colleague, Dr. Richard Quinton. "This was a wonderful coincidence. He told me that this was very interesting as he had a family in Newcastle [England] with three members who had acromegaly or gigantism. I said to him, oh my God, we could study their DNA. I had no doubt this was a genetic disease." Dr. Quinton arranged a study agreement and had the patients' DNA forwarded to Professor Korbonits.

Professor Korbonits' good fortune continued when she started collaborating with an endocrinologist in Chicago, Professor Larry Frohman, who was a pioneer in studying familial acromegaly. When he retired, "I practically took over from him this aspect of this research." She now had a trove of cases that appeared to be genetic in nature.

Professor Korbonits was not the only researcher interested in studying genetic acromegaly and gigantism. Finnish researchers at Helsinki University had been studying familial, or hereditary, pituitary tumors for more than a decade. They suspected that the tumors were genetic in nature when three families in Northern Finland were found to have growth hormone secreting pituitary tumors affecting several family members.[2] In 2004, Dr. Auli Karhu, in the university's Genome Biology department, began to look for a gene mutation that might be responsible for gigantism. Even though the Finnish population is genetically very similar, the task

---

1 Malta is a former Crown Colony of the British Empire and a member of the Commonwealth of Nations.

2 Outi Vierimaa et al., "Pituitary adenoma predisposition caused by germline mutations in the *AIP* gene," *Science* 312, no. 5777 (May 26, 2006): 1228-1230.

was not easy given that there are three billion base pairs that make up the 20,000 genes in human DNA.[3]

Based on analysis of the DNA from the Finnish families, Dr. Karhu and her colleagues located a large region on chromosome 11 that they suspected to be the location for the genetic mutation.[4][5] When they sequenced the *AIP* gene which was in the region that they identified on chromosome 11, they noticed right away that something was wrong. They found the genetic mutation that caused the Finnish patients to develop gigantism: a Gln14Stop mutation on the *AIP* gene.

When their findings were released in 2006, Professor Korbonits thought of the families on her caseload that she suspected of having a genetic form of gigantism. "As soon as the Finnish paper came out, the very first family from Newcastle was sequenced, and we found an *AIP* mutation straight away. That was my family number one. I was extremely excited that this is indeed something which can be identified in patients." Professor Korbonits continued to test patients in her study group and found that some with childhood onset disease and a family history of pituitary tumors had a change in their *AIP* gene. Professor Korbonits steadily found more and more families with *AIP* mutations at different places

--------

3 To understand the difficulty in pinpointing a genetic mutation, it is important to understand DNA. DNA looks like a twisted ladder with the side rails of the ladder made from sugar-phosphate and the rungs of the ladder made up of base pairs bound together by hydrogen bonds. There are four bases--guanine, cytosine, adenine, and thymine—and the entire genetic code is determined by how those four bases are ordered into base pairs on the DNA ladder. A genetic mutation occurs when one or more of the bases are changed or ordered incorrectly, which can lead to an inappropriate code for amino acids, the building blocks of proteins. The wrong code can distort the proteins and cause a disease that is passed down through a family.

4 Monica R. Gadelha et al., "Loss of Heterozygosity on Chromosome 11q13 in Two Families with Acromegaly/Gigantism Is Independent of Mutations of the Multiple Endocrine Neoplasia Type I Gene," *Journal of Clinical Endocrinology and Metabolism* 84 (1999): 249-256.

5 Beatriz S. Soares et al., "Tumor Deletion Mapping on Chromosome 11q13 in Eight Families with Isolated Familial Somatotropinoma and in 15 Sporadic Somatotropinomas," *Journal of Clinical Endocrinology and Metabolism* 90 (2005): 6580-6587.

along the 1000 base pairs found in the *AIP* gene.[6] [7]

Then something caught her eye. She noticed that many of her patients who came from or had family connections to Northern Ireland had a particular *AIP* mutation known as an Arg304Stop mutation. In 2008, a young man with teenage onset acromegaly and his cousin with gigantism, who was originally treated in Belfast, Northern Ireland, walked into her office. She took the cousin's DNA sample and found the Arg304Stop mutation in his DNA that she saw in other patients from Northern Ireland.

It was at this point that her research took a dramatic turn when she recalled a conversation that she had with Professor Besser some 20 years before she studied *AIP* mutations. "I didn't think of it for over 20 years and then it came out like a flash. I just remembered. I said to my colleagues a bit jokingly, I wonder if there could be a link to the Irish Giant in the museum. They just laughed at me, but I took my silly idea quite seriously." When she told me the story, she struggled to explain to me how she made this intuitive leap and remembered Charles Byrne. She may not have understood why she remembered, but all I could think about was how lucky I was that she experienced this bit of scientific serendipity that led her to meet her newest patient, Charles Byrne.

As with any new patient, she began with a review of his medical records. To fit the profile of a patient with a pituitary tumor that causes gigantism due to an *AIP* gene variant, three attributes generally are present: the patient has a hormone secreting tumor, childhood onset of the tumor, and relatives with the same disease. There was no doubt that Charles Byrne

---

6 In about 10% of the cases, pituitary tumors caused by *AIP* gene mutations are also implicated in other excess hormones, such as prolactin. The tumor is then called a prolactinoma.

7 The *AIP* gene is believed to be a tumor suppressor gene in the pituitary gland, so its function is to regulate cell replication and prevent tumor development. Damage to the *AIP* gene increases the likelihood that a benign tumor or adenoma will form on the pituitary gland. The *AIP* gene is approximately 1000 DNA base pairs long and can undergo mutations or changes at any point along the chain of base pairs. Sometimes, a gene variant can be a deletion where part of the gene is missing. Other times it can be an insertion or duplication of base pairs that are abnormal, altering the translation of the message to the correct protein.

had the first attribute: a hormone secreting tumor. He was extremely tall, and his skull showed that he had an enlarged pituitary fossa, prominent jawbone, and large frontal sinuses--all characteristics of someone with a growth hormone secreting tumor on his pituitary gland.

To assess the second attribute, Professor Korbonits looked at the stories from the 18th century that talked about Byrne's great height at a young age, which indicated a childhood onset of his tumor. She also found scientific evidence from x-rays of his wrist bones done by a Swiss neurosurgeon in 1980.[8] She could see that Dr. John Hunter used extra nails and wire on Byrne's wrists when he assembled Byrne's skeleton because his growth plates at the end of his long bones did not fuse before he died when he was 22 years old. "A normal healthy man would stop growing around the age of 18 so if somebody is still growing at the age of 22 that means something is abnormal. That gives an explanation as to why he's so tall: he had lots of growth hormone, and he was able to carry on just growing and growing because his bones did not fuse at the normal time."

To figure out whether he had the third attribute, she needed to find relatives of Charles Byrne who had the disease. She found those relatives in the National Portrait Gallery in London—a gallery with more than 150,000 portraits from the 16th century to the modern day, including sketches and caricatures of local celebrities and oddities created by John Kay in the 18th century. "There is one with Charles Byrne in the middle, and then according to the museum, the two gentlemen standing next to him are his cousins, the Knipe brothers. We can see from Kay's drawing that these distant cousins are twin brothers, and they also have gigantism. We have here three family members who have a very rare disease so this suggests that there must be a genetic condition behind the disease." The Knipe brothers, known as the Gigantic Irish Twins, contributed to Byrne's

---

8 A.M. Landolt and M. Zachmann, "The Irish Giant: New Observations Concerning the Nature of His Ailment," *Lancet* 1, no. 8181 (1980): 1311-1312.

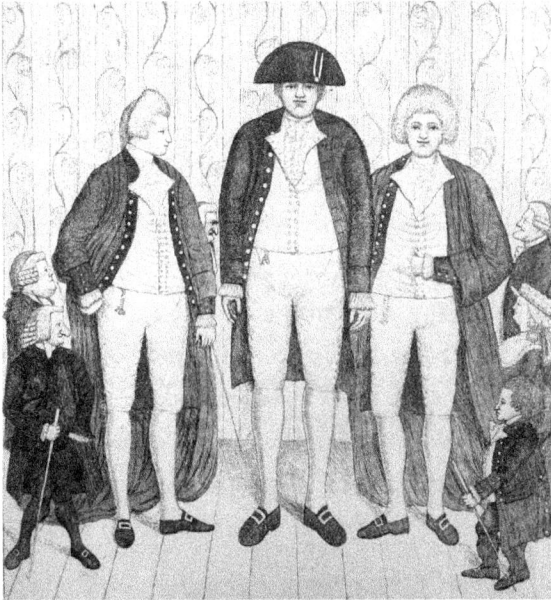

Charles Byrne with the Knipe twins

decline as the most famous Irish giant in London, but in the 21$^{st}$ century, they proved that he had blood relatives with gigantism.

Although it may have seemed far-fetched to her colleagues that a skeleton hanging for more than 200 years in a museum had the same rare genetic disease found in her modern-day research subjects, Professor Korbonits was not deterred by their skepticism. She wrote to the Hunterian Museum with a request to obtain DNA from Byrne's skeleton and permission to examine his bones. They wrote back saying they would discuss her request at their next Board meeting in a few months but reassured her that the museum often provided samples to scientists, especially because genetics offered a novel avenue of study for researchers.

While she was waiting for authorization, she wasted no time and continued with her research and found three more families from Northern Ireland with the same *AIP* mutation. While she knew that they all came from Northern Ireland, she did not know the exact geographic location of each of the families until she began working with Ronan on the documentary, and he showed her where they each lived. "Ronan was a really big help with this when he assisted me to map where the families were coming from, and I started to learn about Northern Irish geography. The village where Charles Byrne was born is not far from the village where Brendan was born, which is about five miles from the Knipe twins, and then I realized that the original family that gave me the first thought regarding *AIP* mutations and Northern Ireland is living just three miles in a line from these villages. So, I thought what is happening here? We got a few more families, and the results were that all of these families were coming from the same narrow geographical area in Northern Ireland where the 18th-century giant came from. They all shared the same abnormal change in the gene, the same mutation, and the same very rare disease."

With the patients' permission, Professor Korbonits continued her research by creating extensive family trees that incorporated information from medical records to document which family members developed acromegaly or gigantism, and when possible, the results of genetic tests for the *AIP* gene. The goal was to figure out how the gene was moving through the bloodline of a family by linking genetics to genealogy.

Genetic researchers use family DNA testing information and their medical records to create a comprehensive medical family pedigree with exact details about how many family members developed the disease, how they are related to each other, and how many family members are carriers of the gene but have not developed the disease. The goal is to figure out how many family members who have the abnormal gene have gone on to develop the disease in proportion to those who do not develop the disease even though they have the mutation. This proportion is called penetrance. For example, Huntington's disease has nearly 100% penetrance, which means that almost all individuals who inherit the gene for Huntington's will get the disease. Other diseases have low penetrance, which means that not everyone who has the defective gene will get the disease. In the case of the Northern Ireland variant of the *AIP* gene, the penetrance is relatively low with between 20-25% of the family members with the genetic mutation developing gigantism.[9]

When I first learned about penetrance, I was struck by how challenging it is for researchers to obtain the necessary information to determine the penetrance of a genetic mutation. Family history is forgotten, medical records can be sketchy or non-existent, and DNA testing is a new technology only available in recent history and at times met with skepticism.

Despite the difficulties, Professor Korbonits pressed on, gathering as much information about each family's history as possible. Oral history and parish records offered vital clues to the identity of family members from generations gone by who might have had acromegaly or gigantism. Old photographs were also a valuable source of information. The trained eye of an endocrinologist can examine vintage photographs of relatives for the key physical characteristics of gigantism—excessive height, facial features, and enlarged hands and feet—to make a diagnosis of gigantism.

In the video of a talk that she gave at the Royal College of Surgeons shortly after her research findings were published, she explained how photographic evidence from one of the families she was studying allowed her to look to the past and find a deceased relative who had gigantism. "The patient's uncle at the age of 18 is standing next an adult lady in this picture. This is not a child. This is an adult lady, and you see the huge difference between the size of the gentleman, and the young woman so it's quite easy to make the diagnosis that this patient with acromegaly had an uncle who also had gigantism."[10]

---

9  Fred Williams, et al., "Clinical Experience in the Screening and Management of a Large Kindred with Familial Isolated Pituitary Adenoma Due to an Aryl Hydrocarbon Receptor Interacting Protein (*AIP*) Mutation," *Journal of Clinical Endocrinology and Metabolism* 99 (2014): 1122-1131.

10  "A Tall Story: Unravelling the Genetics Behind Charles Byrne – 'The Irish Giant,'" The Royal Colleges of Surgeons, Society for Endocrinology, London, November 23, 2011, video, https://youtu.be/IWaPgnk1-Kc.

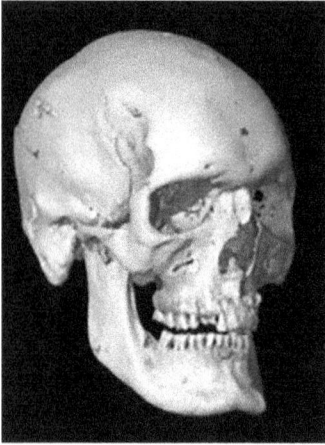

Microcomputer tomography
of Charles Byrne's skull

Months passed as she continued her research. Finally, six months later, the long-awaited reply from the Hunterian Museum arrived, granting her permission to examine Byrne's skeleton and obtain his DNA. She sprang into action. "We took the skull to the Natural History Museum where there is a machine called a microcomputer tomography. We made three-dimensional images from the skull using this machine, and you can see the characteristic features, the thick bones, the very long jawbone, the quite prominent eyebrows, and the huge frontal sinus." The 3-D images confirmed that Byrne had the physical characteristics of a person with acromegaly or gigantism.

Next, she needed to obtain a sample of Byrne's bone to analyze it for his DNA. It was unclear if she would be able to obtain the DNA because of the skeleton's age and condition, given that Dr. Hunter boiled Byrne's bones in an acidic solution, likely degrading its DNA. She consulted with a specialist who recommended that she take a tooth sample, so she asked Mr. Martyn Cooke, Head of Conservation at the Hunterian Museum to remove a tooth from both sides of the lower jaw. "These two teeth which were removed were very precious samples. I wanted the DNA to be extracted in an expert laboratory, so I contacted the paleogenetics laboratory in Germany which specialized in ancient DNA."

Obtaining DNA from ancient bone is a painstaking process demanding a high level of expertise and sufficient time to complete the complex analysis. Professor Korbonits waited patiently for the results to see if her hypothesis about Byrne's DNA would hold true.

Eight weeks later, the results arrived. They confirmed Professor Korbonits' hypothesis: Charles Byrne's DNA had the same Arg304Stop

*AIP* gene variant found on chromosome 11 as the modern-day families she was studying. This made it very likely, but still not 100% certain, that the Irish families she was studying were related to each other and to Charles Byrne. To confirm the relationship, more testing was needed.

To answer the question as to whether they were related to each other, she needed to look more closely at the DNA surrounding the *AIP* gene. Professor Korbonits explained, "The length of the identical region around the gene variant shows how closely people are related to each other. The longer the identical stretch of the DNA region, the closer the relatives are to the subjects that we are studying. To test the similarity of the regions around the *AIP* gene, we use DNA markers called microsatellites. Siblings, for example, have huge sections of DNA with identical microsatellites, showing that they are closely related. If the same sample of DNA was compared to a distant cousin or great-great-great grandparent, the section of DNA with identical microsatellites would be much smaller. It will still, however, be detectable, compared to non-relatives whose section of this DNA will not be similar at all. This is the concept that we used to prove that Byrne is related to Brendan as well as all the other Irish patients with the Arg304Stop *AIP* mutation."

By looking very closely at the Chromosome 11q13 location (the location of the *AIP* gene), she found the same unique pattern of microsatellites in the DNA samples of the Irish families in her study, including Brendan and Charles Byrne. Professor Korbonits noted that, "the only possibility for this to happen is if these families had a common ancestor somewhere in the past so that meant that they were related to each other. The living patients may not necessarily know each other, but we know from this genetic study that they all are distant cousins of each other." Her 21st-century patients were now linked to her 18th-century one.

But could she go back even further in time? How long ago did the first person to have this mutation live? To get the answer to that question, she asked her colleagues in the University College to do a statistical genetic analysis of the Northern Irish families in her study using what is known as the coalescent theory. The coalescent theory is a mathematical model used in population genetics to trace a gene variant back to a single common ancestor. By analyzing genetic data from the Human Genome Diversity Project (HapMap), researchers estimate when a gene mutation first appeared by figuring out roughly how many generations ago it happened. Her colleagues determined, using all the Irish families identified with the gene mutation until 2017, that the common ancestor (or mutation founder) lived between 51-200 generations. Assuming one generation is about 25 years long, that means that the common ancestor lived an astounding 1,275–5,000 years ago.[11]

The determination that the common ancestor who first had the defective gene that caused gigantism lived hundreds if not thousands of years ago raises even more fascinating questions. Could this genetic variant that causes gigantism in patients in Northern Ireland explain the prevalence of Irish giant mythology and legend in the northernmost areas of the island of Ireland? Could the stories of the Fenian warriors and their giant leader Fionn Mac Cumhaill of the Giant's Causeway fame have a basis in truth? Could the many giant graves found in County Tyrone documented in the Placenames Database of Ireland point to real giants who once lived in the area and suffered from gigantism linked to an *AIP* gene variant? Could mythology and legends from thousands of years ago be validated through modern DNA analysis?

Professor Korbonits' use of statistical analysis not only allowed her to peer into the past, but statistics also gave her a tool to figure out how many people living today might be carrying the giant gene. Even though her colleagues needed to consider a variety of mitigating factors, such as early death, reduced fertility (a common symptom of gigantism), and historic

11  Harvinder S. Radian, et al., "Increased Population Risk of AIP-Related Acromegaly and Gigantism in Ireland," *Human Mutation* 38 (2017): 78-85.

events such as wars, they believed they could come up with an estimate. They determined that the range was between 90 and 5175 people alive today with the mutation with a range of 18 to 1035 of them going on to develop gigantism.

When I heard the estimated number of how many people today might have the genetic mutation and how many would likely develop the disease, I was heartened by the small number, but I quickly remembered that the impact of having the mutation can be immense for an individual family. I knew just how important it is to know that the defective gene is in a family's pedigree. It gives the family a valuable tool, a way to track the giant gene through the family and find the children who may have the defective gene before they suffer the devastating effects of having a pituitary tumor and undiagnosed gigantism.

In the spring of 2010, Professor Korbonits and her team of 17 researchers submitted the findings found in "*AIP* Mutation in Pituitary Adenomas in the 18^th Century and Today" for review by the *New England Journal of Medicine*. Five sentences in the journal article summed them up:

> Gigantism results when a growth hormone–secreting pituitary adenoma is present before epiphyseal fusion. In 1909, when Harvey Cushing examined the skeleton of an Irish patient who lived from 1761 to 1783, he noted an enlarged pituitary fossa. We extracted DNA from the patient's teeth and identified a germline mutation in the aryl hydrocarbon–interacting protein gene (AIP). Four contemporary Northern Irish families who presented with gigantism, acromegaly, or prolactinoma have the same mutation and haplotype associated with the mutated gene. Using coalescent theory, we infer

that these persons share a common ancestor who lived about 57 to 66 generations earlier.[1213]

These five simple declarative sentences represented more than six years of in-depth research, cutting-edge techniques, and detailed analysis. The research encompassed endocrinology, genetics, genomics, paleogenetics, natural history, evolutionary biology, and biomedical science with input from researchers from England, Northern Ireland, Germany, and Sweden. A cohort of 140 families were considered in the overall analysis before the researchers zeroed in on four modern Irish families and Charles Byrne to be the focus of the paper. For each of the four families, researchers obtained oral family history and artifacts such as photographs, medical records, when available, did clinical examinations, and gathered DNA samples from as many living family members as possible to create detailed family pedigrees. It took dogged determination, incredible attention to detail, and excellent detective skills to accumulate the data needed for the findings summarized in those five simple sentences.

There was still one final hurdle to pass—the approval of the submitted article for publication. As Professor Korbonits waited for the approval, Ronan contacted her to let her know that the documentary was ready for release. "His film was ready in the summer, and I told him you cannot release it until the paper comes out, so he sat on a ready film which is quite something for a filmmaker, but he did it. So that is really something and speaks to the type of guy he is. I was right to trust him." The trust that they developed allowed both to benefit. Ronan had a much deeper story than he could have possibly imagined when he started filming, and Professor

---

12  Harvinder S. Chahal, et al., "AIP Mutation in Pituitary Adenomas in the 18th Century and Today," *The New England Journal of Medicine* 8 (2011), 1.

13  A few years after the paper was published, Professor Korbonits extended the mathematical analysis using the coalescent theory to not just 4 but 18 families , which revealed that the common ancestor lived about 102 generations ago or approximately 2550 years ago.

Korbonits had a film that captured the story of her research to the benefit of her patients affected by gigantism.

Six months later, in January 2011, Professor Korbonits' paper was published. Four days after publication, BBC-Northern Ireland broadcast *Charles Byrne: the Irish Giant/an Fathach Éireannach*. The Irish language station TG4 aired the documentary five days later. To date, it has been viewed more than 166,000 times on YouTube.

# CHAPTER 6

# EXPLORING THE BRANCHES

*I feel like hiding in a burrow/There I'd have no fears, have no worries.*
*I feel like jumping off a cliff/Then I'd have no life to live.*
*But I want no sorrow or for me to die/So what can I do but cry.*
*I will go and weep a while/Life has to get better.*

—NIAMH FEENEY from "My Life"
County Sligo, Ireland

As the pandemic wore on, I was surprised at the stark contrast between my real life and my online life. My day-to-day existence felt limited and constricted. It revolved around the constant worry of how best to avoid people and how to assess the safety of any environment other than my house or my car. Fully masked, armed with hand sanitizer, I ventured into a store as long as the goal was to get in and out as quickly as possible.

However, as soon as I sat in my office chair, flipped on my computer, and the monitor came to life, relief washed over me as I dived into a virtual world far removed from the pandemic around me. With a click of the mouse, I was in Northern Ireland talking with Brendan. Another click, I was researching the lives of Byrne or Dr. Hunter in the Internet Archive. Online videos, podcasts, and websites about genetics, endocrinology, mythology, genealogy, and medical research were all at my fingertips. I learned to embrace my online life.

I grew to appreciate how intimate Zoom calls felt when I was face-to-face with another person with no distractions. I particularly felt this bond when I met online with Brendan's relatives who were also affected

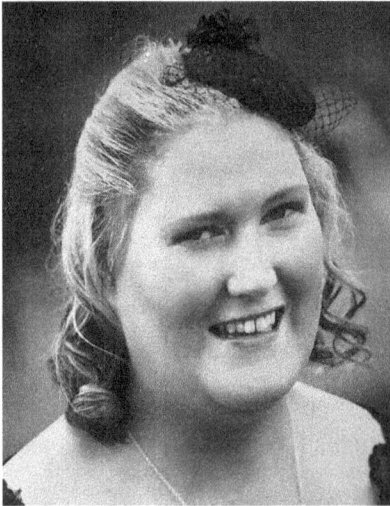

Niamh Feeney

by gigantism, so I was very interested in meeting Brendan's cousin Niamh. I saw her in Ronan's documentary when he filmed her at home in County Sligo in the west of Ireland. Brendan first met Niamh in 1994. A friend told him about her 13-year-old niece Niamh who was growing much faster than other girls and asked Brendan to travel to County Sligo to meet her and share his experiences with having gigantism. Brendan remembered her as being quite shy and reluctant to talk

with him. When Brendan offered to connect me with Niamh, I jumped at the chance and scheduled a video chat with her.

When Niamh appeared on my computer screen, the shy teenager that Brendan remembered was now a confident 40-year-old woman still living in her childhood home in Grange, not far from the beaches of Mullaghmore. As I looked at her on my computer screen while we chatted, the lively and outgoing Niamh struck me as someone who has made peace with the challenges that she faced, despite the disappointments in her life derailed by a pituitary tumor. Her story and diagnostic odyssey were heartbreaking.

She talked fondly about her childhood and her dream of going to college to become a teacher like her mother. School was a haven for her, filled with kind friends and patient teachers. Around the age of 11, she started to grow quite rapidly, but it wasn't until a year later when she was unable to read the classroom blackboard that her mother became concerned. A visit to the eye doctor upended Niamh's life.

The local doctor determined that she was unable to see clearly out of her left eye, but the answer as to why took several doctor appointments. Niamh remembers her diagnostic journey. "I couldn't see that well with my left eye when I was 12. I went to a few eye doctors in Sligo, but they couldn't see anything wrong with my eyes, so they sent me up to Mater Hospital in Dublin to have a visual field studies test. They could see the problem was behind my eye, so I had a CT scan. That's when they found the tumor." The pituitary tumor was pressing on her optic nerve, causing her to have decreased vision. Bloodwork revealed the excess growth hormone caused by the tumor, resulting in her rapid growth.

She now knew the cause of her excessive growth and vision loss. But her journey didn't stop there. Her care was transferred to Beaumont Hospital, one of Ireland's top hospitals and an academic partner of Ireland's Royal College of Surgeons. She told me that she remembered little about her first meeting with Brendan. "I knew about Brendan, but I didn't know we were related until much later. He was just my uncle's friend at that time." Niamh was scheduled for surgery in hopes of removing the tumor, restoring her vision, and alleviating her excess growth hormone. Maybe they caught the tumor in time.

Niamh remembered that hopes ran high when she left Mater Hospital and arrived at Beaumont Hospital to prepare for her surgery. Her mother and some of her relatives were on hand to help with her transfer. "When we got to the children's ward at Beaumont, we all thought it was lovely. Cartoon characters were all over the walls. The nurses were all lovely too, and a doctor came round and told us that we could go home for the weekend." Niamh was delighted to get a break from being in a hospital before the actual surgery. The next day Niamh's uncle Raymond took her home.

"I had the best weekend of my teenage life. All of my friends were over. I was the center of attention, just what I'd wished for, and I loved it. I wished it would last forever."

After the idyllic weekend, Niamh returned to Beaumont Hospital, and the next day she underwent pituitary surgery to remove the tumor. "At half eight, the surgeons took me to the [operating] theatre. When mum and dad could no longer go with me, I put on a brave face and said I was ok. Inside, I was shouting at them to come. I didn't want to be on my own in there, but I knew they couldn't come. I remember a young lady giving me an injection and telling me to count from 10 down to 1. I only managed to make it to 9."

Unfortunately, unexpected complications occurred. "My mum's face was the first I saw when I woke. I smiled and tried to say 'hi,' but it couldn't come out of my mouth. I just thought I was tired and fell back asleep. The next day, a nurse asked me my name. I couldn't say it. She asked me where I was. I knew that I was in the hospital after an operation, but the words just would not come out right. I was frustrated. Mum and Dad came up to me later that day and told me that I had had a stroke. I had lost the ability to talk. I could not move my right arm and hand, and my right leg and foot were paralyzed." Niamh was only 13 years old.

In addition to learning that she had a stroke, Niamh also found out that the operation was not a complete success. "I had the operation to remove the tumor, but they couldn't remove all of it because it was too close to other tissues and the doctors were afraid of damaging something." The news was bitterly disappointing. "I had a row of staple stitches where my hair met my forehead from ear to ear. When I looked at myself for the first time since the operation, I felt I was the laughingstock of the ward. All the left-hand side of my face was drooped down. It wasn't equal to the right-hand side. I just wanted to hide."

Niamh faced a life far different than the one she hoped for prior to the surgery. Rather than rejoining her classmates and continuing her life, she spent the next year in Dún Laoghaire at the National Rehabilitation Hospital learning to walk and talk again. "Physio is where I relearned how to use my leg. It was tough work. In speech therapy, I started on the basic three-letter words like bat, pat, bin, and sin. I used to get mixed up with my Bs and Ds, and I couldn't pronounce the sound of the letter S, but I got there. I learnt how to write with my left hand."

When she left Dún Laoghaire to return to school after a year, her right hand was paralyzed, she walked with a limp, and talking was difficult and slow. "When I came into my classroom, a big cheer was heard from everybody. All my classmates came up and hugged me. I just loved it. Getting to know them all again; it was great. But then schoolwork started, and I was lost." Her classwork proved to be far too challenging after the trauma of the surgery and a year's absence for rehabilitation. Her mother suggested that she repeat the school year, and Niamh agreed. "It was a struggle to keep up with all the work. Sometimes I would even fall asleep going home in the car. I'd be that wrecked. But I managed it with a lot of help from all the teachers, friends, and family."

Because the surgery was not a complete success, the remaining tumor still affected her pituitary gland, and she continued to have excess growth hormone. She grew even taller despite the intervention, so the doctors recommended radiotherapy. After a year of intensive speech and physical therapy and a full course of radiotherapy, Niamh went home still suffering from excess growth hormone and the other negative effects of having a pituitary tumor.

Brendan entered the picture and offered to help Niamh in any way possible. "At this point I went to see her again. I was shocked to see the damage done to this tender, sensitive young lady. Her mother Marianna asked if I could liaise with St. Bartholomew's Hospital to get her treatment. I contacted Professor Mike Besser who agreed to treat her if the Irish Health Service provided funding to the UK National Health Service. It was difficult because they are two separate health care systems, but the funding was secured." At the time, Brendan had a small apartment near London that he used for business, so Marianna and Niamh stayed with him during the testing to assess her condition.

Brendan also found out that Niamh's mother was quite ill. "While Marianna and I were waiting for Niamh one day, Marianna told me that she was suffering from terminal cancer and did not have long to live." Although her husband and family were aware of her situation, she decided to keep it from Niamh. Brendan promised Marianna that she could rely on him to see Niamh's treatment through, even in her absence.

With Professor Besser and Brendan's help, Niamh received further treatment, undergoing surgery and radiotherapy once again. The tumor was now only a remnant, with no active cells in it. But the effects of the tumor continued to haunt her. "I was wrecked in secondary school. I had to stay back a year because I missed so much school. I was so shy and nervous. Everybody was staring at me, the giant, hunchback girl with a major limp. I hated myself. The girls in my class and year were so nice to me. The teachers were too, but I hated secondary school. It was far too hard. I spent every night crying, asking Mum why God hated me so much and why God did this to me."

In 1999, shortly after Niamh's final treatment, Niamh's mother passed away from cancer. "My tumor stopped growing, thank God, but Mum's cancer was worse. I blame myself for her dying. She put so much of her hope, strength and energy into me getting better; she had none left for herself." Not only did Niamh need to learn how to navigate her life after the damage caused by the surgery, but she also had to learn how to live without her mother by her side. Niamh was 18 years old.

After hearing Niamh's story about her diagnosis and treatment, I asked her what happened after secondary school and her mother's death. Although she was unable to complete her leaving certifications for school at the time, she was able to enter a program for people with disabilities that offered her a lifeline to continue learning and to help her move forward with her life. She took computer classes, enjoyed a creative writing class where she wrote stories filled with elves and fairies, and worked as an information officer while in the program. She was elated when she learned to drive a car that she called her "little red beauty," a Mitsubishi Colt modified to accommodate her right-side paralysis with an accelerator on the left side and a knob on the steering wheel to help with one-handed driving. She later took her certifications over again and passed.

Niamh and Brendan met once again, but this time it was clear to both that they were related. Shortly after Brendan discovered that he had the *AIP* mutation, he recommended that Niamh be evaluated for the giant gene because of their family connection. As expected, given her history of having the *AIP* mutation in her family pedigree, she tested positive for the mutation. She now had the answer to why she developed the pituitary tumor that changed her life.

During the shooting of the Charles Byrne documentary, Ronan and Brendan traveled to Niamh's home in Grange to film Brendan and Niamh as they spent time together and shared their stories. Afterwards, they headed northwest to the crescent shaped Mullaghmore beach that wraps the bay with sand dunes with the Tievebaun and Truskmore mountains in the distance. The two of them walked along the sand, isolated from others but joined together by a common diagnosis and a genetic mutation that impacted their lives.

During my time on Zoom with Niamh, I asked her about what she learned from the challenges she faced given her gigantism diagnosis and treatment. Her answer showed her resolve to move forward with her life with determination and dignity. "I am 6 foot 4 inches (193 cm) and 41 years old now. I do think every day about what my life would have been like if I hadn't had the tumor. I do get really tired throughout the day, so I can't work a full-time job. I am still living at home with my Dad because I can't afford to rent a house. I wanted to be married and have children. I always wanted to become a primary school teacher, like my Mum, but that never surfaced. But I do think, yes, I had the tumor, and yes, I had a stroke, but what if I had never regained speech or learnt how to walk again? There are always positives to negatives. I wouldn't have known what it was like to have the gigantism gene. I have met so many people because of this gene and this stroke. Who doesn't wish, at least once in a lifetime, they were someone else. But I am happy. I am content. I am me."

Niamh's story is at once tragic and inspiring. It is inspiring to witness her strength as a young girl overcoming the trauma of surgery and a stroke. I admire how, as an adult, she has learned to accept her life despite the setbacks she experienced. Unfortunately, the tragedy of her diagnostic and treatment journey, as her mother helped her search for a diagnosis and effective treatment, is a hallmark for patients who have a rare disease such as gigantism. For Niamh, it took several eye doctors and a referral to a Dublin hospital before she received her diagnosis. Her treatment plan spanned two countries, two surgeries, two courses of radiotherapy, and months of rehabilitation.

In my case, it took 12 years until I got a diagnosis. I have often questioned how I was hospitalized for extensive testing twice when I was diagnosed with rheumatic fever and then mononucleosis as a teenager, yet the doctors never noticed the clear acromegaly symptoms I was exhibiting. I wonder how different my life would have been if I had known that I had the *AIP* gene mutation and been monitored for symptoms of gigantism. What would it have been like to have a body without a pituitary tumor and unaffected by excess growth hormone?

After I waved goodbye to Niamh and clicked "leave meeting" to sign off Zoom, I sat for a while just looking out of my window, reflecting on what we had shared. I was grateful that Niamh spoke so candidly with me about her life, particularly when she talked about what it was like to be with people who do not have physical challenges.

I could really relate to what Niamh said when she recalled how painful it was to have the other children comment on and tease her about her appearance as she was growing up. While the rude stares and unsettling comments from children can be written off as mere juvenile curiosity, the sidelong glances and unwelcome remarks by adults weighed even heavier. I thought back to something Niamh said in the documentary that really stuck with me. "People in town would give me a second look. I just hate it. I think, 'What have you got? I'll give you a second look and see how you like it.' I know they don't mean to do it, but even small children when I am queuing for something, the children come up to me and look up. And I think, just disappear."[1]

My conversation with Niamh also reminded me of how gangly and awkward I felt when I was young and how that made me want to hide away from others. I felt alienated from those around me. Even something as simple as buying shoes became an ordeal when I couldn't find shoes that fit. Niamh mentioned how she needed to hunch to get through doorways that are too short. Not being able to walk comfortably through a physical space or find shoes that fit were symbols of how we were not in sync with the others around us.

I later came across a chapter in the book *Body Image: A Handbook of Theory, Research, and Clinical Practice* that captured what I felt so deeply when I was around other people, and what Niamh shared with me during our Zoom conversation. "In contrast to the anonymity enjoyed by people with an unremarkable appearance, a person who is visibly different becomes a focus of usually unwanted attention, including staring, comments, and questions…Others demonstrate nonverbal and verbal behavior reflecting reactions of aversion, surprise, or discomfort."[2] With a body different from others, we cannot be invisible.

---

1 Ronan McCloskey, *Charles Byrne: the Irish Giant/an Fathach Éireannach,* video, BBC Northern Ireland, 2011, https://www.youtube.com/watch?v=xLA-KZ7sBLg.

2 Nichola Rumsey, "Body Image and Congenital Conditions with Visible Differences," in *Body Image: A Handbook of Theory, Research, and Clinical Practice,* ed. Thomas F. Cash and Thomas Pruzinsky (New York: The Guilford Press), 229.

Even now that the tumor is gone, the ghost of the pituitary tumor still resides in us, coloring our world simply because of everything we have gone through because we had a pituitary tumor. Niamh, Brendan, and I, along with others who share our diagnosis, have seen the essence of the tumor and know its nature. Though tiny, the tumor was powerful enough to change our faces and our bodies and disrupt our lives. It was random, striking us but not our other relatives who also had the same genetic mutation. It was sly, lurking during our childhoods, waiting years to be discovered. It was relentless, continuing to affect our lives long after the tumor was gone.

# CHAPTER 7

# THE PROMISE OF
# CASCADE TESTING

When I found out I had the genetic mutation, Professor Korbonits encouraged me to create a comprehensive family tree in the hope of tracing the gene through my family to test and identify anyone at risk of developing gigantism. I began working on getting my three adult children evaluated. I knew the importance of having my cousins screened, but I was unsure of how to convince them to get tested. I barely knew my cousins and was not sure how to approach them. DNA testing is a sensitive topic with many people concerned about how the information is used. Unlike the ease and low cost of getting DNA results through a company like Ancestry.com or 23 and Me for genealogy information, DNA testing for a medical condition related to a genetic mutation can be expensive and difficult to obtain in the United States because of our healthcare system. Getting an appointment with a geneticist, obtaining the proper referral, and getting prior authorization for an unusual DNA test are barriers to obtaining care.

I asked Brendan how his family reacted to getting tested and how the process worked for him and his family. As Brendan told me about his family, I realized that his family illustrates how cascade testing works and the benefits of getting relatives screened for a genetic mutation.

# IN SEARCH OF GIANTS

Cascade testing is a tool that geneticists use to shine a light on a defective gene discovered through genetic testing, identify the carriers of the gene in the family, and trace that genetic mutation through a person's family tree or pedigree. The process is systematic, beginning with a known carrier and moving outward from that person. First, the immediate family members—parents, children, and siblings—of the carrier are tested. Next, the immediate family of the those in the first round who had positive results are then tested. Further rounds of testing occur to find all individuals who might be at risk.

Because Brendan had the *AIP* mutation, all seven of his siblings and his two children were at risk with each of them having a 50% chance of having the genetic mutation. (His parents were not alive, so they could not be tested.) Neither of his children were found to have the mutation, so no further testing was required for their immediate families. All his siblings underwent genetic testing, and three of the seven tested positive for the mutation. The other siblings tested negative, so no additional testing of their genetic lines was necessary. For the three siblings that tested positive, the testing "cascaded" to the next generation, with their children having the same 50% chance of having the mutation. One of the siblings had four children, with three of them testing positive, and the second sibling had three children, with one of them testing positive.

The testing then cascaded to the next generation and the children of the four children who tested positive were then tested. The results revealed that three children from the next generation were positive. Although none of the family members at this point were known to have a pituitary tumor, Brendan's siblings and their families had the advantage of knowing their status and receiving appropriate monitoring going forward.

For Brendan's third sibling who tested positive for the mutation, his brother Aidan, cascade testing proved to be invaluable for the health of his children. When Aidan first learned about Brendan's positive test for the mutation and was asked to be screened for the gene, he was eager to participate and learn more about the impact on his family. "I got to learn about the disease and how it affects the people who are carriers even if they don't appear to have any problem. I got the benefit of [Professor Korbonits' research] reflected back on my family when I found out I was a carrier. You don't realize at the time that somebody close to you is going to be affected as well. You are glad that you actually got involved in the whole thing."

Cascade testing revealed that all three of Aidan's children had the genetic mutation. When Aidan's daughter Laura received her positive test results, she underwent more testing to detect any endocrine problems. The additional testing altered the trajectory of her life. Despite never living in the geographic hotspot, given she was born in England, her genetic heritage remained with her. Her clinical screening revealed that she had an undiagnosed pituitary tumor.

When Brendan told me about Laura and a bit of her story, I was eager to connect with her and hear the details of what happened to her before and after her diagnosis. Once again, Zoom allowed me to reach across the ocean to connect with her in her home in Bromley, to the south of London. When she popped up on my computer screen, right away, I felt a kinship with her as she greeted me, and we began chatting about the challenges she faced before and after she found out about the genetic mutation that caused her tumor. I could see the lingering effects of having gigantism reflected in her face, which only made me feel more comfortable with her as we shared our stories.

Not only was I interested in hearing her story and her diagnostic journey, I was very curious to find out why her diagnosis was delayed for so many years despite having a close family relative, her uncle Brendan, who also had a pituitary tumor. To learn the details, we started with her childhood, and her earliest experiences with symptoms that she now knew were related to the tumor. "My mum and dad met in London, which is where I was born and where I still live. My earliest memory is the nickname I had where I grew up when the children called me "BFG" [from Roald Dahl's children's book *The BFG* or big friendly giant]. They always said it in a nice way, so I didn't take it as offensive. I was taller than everyone else including the boys, so that was one of the names that they called me."

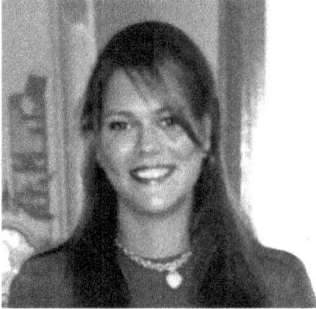

Laura, age 23

She went on to tell me about her teenage years. "My other memories are as a teenager when I was so incredibly shy and self-conscious, and I realized I was not as feminine looking as my friends. I also noticed how my shoe size kept going up unlike my friends. The other thing I've noticed is how few photographs I have from that time. A couple of my friends were really snap-happy, always bringing their cameras, but I really disliked having my photo taken and told my friends to take down photographs on Facebook because I was shocked by what I looked like. I just thought I wasn't aging well. I am still self-conscious. My face feels like it's twice the size of everyone else's. I don't think I look like that in all photos, but I'm always aware." I understood exactly what she meant. I hated to have photographs taken when I was a teenager. To this day, I avoid having my picture taken, and when I see a photograph of myself, I always focus on how big my head looks in comparison to others. I feel very uncomfortable with my image.

The changes in her body were so subtle that even those closest to her had trouble seeing that it was a disease process taking place, not just the changes that come from a teen going through puberty. "When I was waiting for the results of the testing, I just knew I had it from all the things I'd been saying over the years. Like, I'd say to my mum, my nose is spreading. My nose is getting really big. My mum said, 'Well, if you look in the mirror long enough, you're bound to find fault' but I could see it in the photographs. I remember another time—this was all when I was in my 20s—my dad said, 'your voice is breaking.' I thought, it is? But girls' voices don't break. So, there were all these little things, these clues. They were always there." She was much taller than her peers and was getting taller as her height approached six feet (183 cm).

By her late twenties, the undetected tumor continued to impact her health as symptoms associated with gigantism became more overt and more damaging. "I had carpal tunnel syndrome and always had pain in my arms. When the doctors asked me about headaches when I was diagnosed, I told them no but what I did have was a searing pain in my left eye. It felt like someone was poking me in the back of my eye. My husband kept telling me to go to the doctor for it. I also told my dentist about a loud clunk in my left jaw every time I opened to eat something like an apple. It clunked, not just a little bit, and anyone sitting near me noticed. He told me that it was just a severe case of teeth grinding." The truth was that it was another symptom of acromegaly.

As the Holland family continued to undergo genetic screening, Laura became more and more convinced that she had a pituitary tumor. "I think I was one of the last to go for testing even though my dad kept saying that I had to go. But I was in my 20s, and I didn't understand the importance until I started looking into it and learned about the symptoms. I could see that my face had changed, and I have photos of me with my oldest brother Bernard who's six foot one (185 cm). He's a very big man, probably 18 stone (252 lb/114.3 kg). And when you look at our faces, mine is much bigger. At this point, he was a bigger, heavier man, but my face was so much bigger. At my first appointment with Dr. Korbonits and the clinical geneticist Dr. Kumar, I noticed them looking at each other, and when I looked at all the symptoms, everything fell into place. I knew I had it, and it all made sense."

At this point, Laura had not yet received a diagnosis because more testing was necessary to confirm what the doctors were suspecting. Laura remembers returning for five or six appointments as the evidence related to her medical condition accumulated. "My brother was going through testing as well, and I think they only called him back once to have an MRI, so I knew that something was going on."

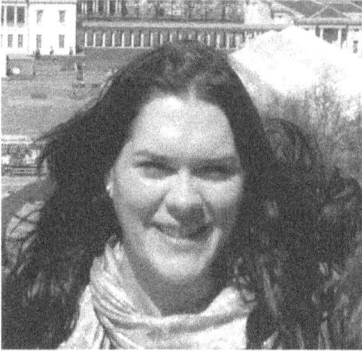

Laura, age 30, 5 months before surgery

Finally, she received her diagnosis. She was positive for the *AIP* mutation, and she had a pituitary tumor as she suspected. It was a macroadenoma that was two centimeters or the size of a cherry tomato. It was pushing on her pituitary on the left, causing the pain in her eye. "My experience with puberty was different from yours. It started later when I was 13. Professor Korbonits thinks that I may have had the beginnings of gigantism then based on my height compared to my female cousins. I'm tallest at 5 feet 10 inches (177 cm). It might be that the puberty hormones superseded the growth hormone, and the tumor lay dormant until my twenties when the physical changes became visible. Although I'm not Brendan's height, Professor Korbonits believes my height is not necessarily a natural height. She says that two or three inches of additional growth are probably due to the growth hormone. She also told me that it might be difficult to have children. That floored me because we were starting to think about having a family."

The cascade testing that Laura's extended family experienced was a success. It not only identified the carriers in the family, but also led to the detection of her undiagnosed pituitary tumor, which caused her symptoms. Her medical team developed a treatment plan to control the excess growth hormone and maintain her fertility. "I had transsphenoidal surgery in 2012 to remove the tumor. They wanted me to go back on the lanreotide injections that suppress growth hormone. I started to take lanreotide when I was first diagnosed. I was adamant that I really wanted to start a family, so they didn't put me back on that. Two years later, I had my first daughter, and two years after that my second daughter. Our family was complete, so I started back on the lanreotide. I still have residual tumor next to my pituitary, but because I am being monitored, I won't need surgery ever again."

For Laura, the future is bright. Cascade testing identified her as having the defective gene and a tumor, which led to an effective treatment and monitoring plan. This allowed her to have children and manage the effects of her residual tumor. "I don't think there will be any surprises, and if there is, I still might do gamma knife radiation. I have only noticed changes when I come off the lanreotide injections and the growth hormone goes up. During Covid lockdown, I missed some injections, and I noticed my shoes were becoming tight. I'm happy to be monitored through my blood testing and MRIs, and I feel good."

Laura made a point of telling me about one woman she met while she was going through treatment whose diagnostic journey was far different from hers. The woman's story reminded Laura of how fortunate she was to get a diagnosis through the cascade testing process. "When I was in the waiting room at Barts, I used to regularly see a woman. At the time, she was probably in her early 50s. She was only recently diagnosed with acromegaly. She was in and out of the hospital multiple times and had many surgeries, such as carpal tunnel surgery. Carpal tunnel is a symptom of acromegaly, but the surgeons didn't notice that she had acromegaly. Finally, she moved and got a different doctor who trained at Barts. When he looked at her record, he knew right away that she might have acromegaly and referred her for testing. She had gone undiagnosed and without treatment all those years, which led to those unnecessary surgeries."

Next, Laura turned her attention to her two daughters. It was time for them to be tested to check their status for the *AIP* mutation. Each of them individually had a 50/50 chance of having the faulty gene. Both were found to be carriers. "So, they have appointments at the Royal London Hospital every year for monitoring. They have tests to check their hormone levels and have their height and weight measured." Each girl has roughly a 25% chance of developing a pituitary tumor due to being a carrier of the gene.

I asked her the obvious question. Was she worried about them? "I hope that it doesn't manifest right away. I do notice that it's my older daughter that tends to get the comments, like when she goes back to school from the summer holidays. People always say how she's gotten really tall, that she's shot up. So that triggers me a bit. But I see the other children, and they are growing too, and I know my daughter is within range because she is being monitored. She will eventually have to have an MRI, and that worries me a bit, but I know that there's no point in worrying just yet."

I went on to ask whether it was worth the stress and worry that goes along with testing and monitoring. Her answer was a resounding yes. "I'm really, really happy. I know that she's in safe hands and that the doctors are aware of what she needs. I do worry for what may happen in the future. But I think it's reassuring that she is being supervised. If anything strange happens, then they will be on top of it. I'd rather be in the know and understand what is going on than not. The alternative of not knowing is far worse."

Laura commented on the value of having her extended family tested. "I think it has helped. Because we all knew Brendan and knew that he's had these health issues. For all that time, everyone thought he was an isolated case, but now we know it's genetic. All my dad's brothers and sisters have been tested, so we know who the carriers are. All the carriers' children have been tested, so we know who is at risk. My brother is a carrier, and because his children were tested, we know whether his children are carriers. Everyone's very keen. Everyone's very aware. How I explain it is in our family, the mutation is not rare. We can all be carriers and not know it. It is the manifestation of the tumor that is rare, so we need to know who is carrying the gene and hasn't manifested the disease."

Her father Aidan agreed. Despite Brendan having a pituitary tumor and gigantism, he didn't realize that his own daughter had a pituitary tumor and symptoms of excess growth hormone because her symptoms were so different than his brother's. "I didn't know that the symptoms she had were related to what Brendan had. It's fortunate that things happened the way that they did. [Professor Korbonits] was the driving force behind that. It was fortunate we have the technology. Twenty or thirty years ago they didn't have the technology. They wouldn't have been able to identify what was happening. It shows how the testing works as it tracks the family. Laura was still affected because of how it is carried through the family. But, when you know the disease is there, monitoring is the easy part. It's easy to get the blood test or any of the tests that tell the medical people what is actually happening. They know what to look for it in the person."

The process for getting the genetic testing done in the UK National Health Service was straightforward with no cost to the patients. Brendan's family knew about the tumor's effect on Brendan, and family members saw the value of getting the testing done. I was eager to find out what cascade testing would reveal about my family.

By looking at my family tree, I knew that my mother, grandmother, and great-grandfather were carriers, but none of them developed gigantism. Still, they passed the mutant gene on to me. It was clear that the disease of gigantism could skip many generations before someone developed the disease. I knew from the research that if someone has the mutation, they will most likely develop the tumor between the ages of 4 and 30. My children were old enough that it was unlikely that they would develop a tumor, but I was still worried that they were carriers and felt guilty that I might have passed the mutation on to them. To find out about my children, they just had to do the DNA test and hope they were lucky enough to avoid inheriting the defective gene.

My oldest son Emmett recently married and was planning to start a family. Could he be a carrier of the genetic mutation? How would the discovery that my acromegalic gigantism was a genetic disease impact him and his children? He took the test. It was an anxious six weeks while we waited to see his result. It was negative, and I was elated. I did not pass it on to him, so none of his descendants would get the defective gene. Next up was my daughter Wren. Once again, after a few uneasy weeks, I was able to let out a sigh of relief when her result was negative as well. That left my son Alexander. I sent off his completed test kit and hoped for the best.

By this point, the difference between obtaining the DNA testing under the American healthcare system and the National Health Service in the UK became very clear. There were four of us that needed to be tested. Each one of us had a different configuration of health insurance systems dictating how we could obtain the DNA test and how much the testing would cost us out-of-pocket. There were four insurance systems involved: Medicare and Cigna private insurance for me, Blue Cross employer-based insurance for my older son, Medicare and Medicaid for my younger son, and a different type of Cigna for my daughter. While my three children were able to go to the same geneticist through a video visit, they all had to get different prior authorizations from their insurance company to have that visit, and we each paid a different amount for the same test, ranging from zero to $350.

Once again, it took about six weeks for Alexander's results to come back. But this time our luck didn't hold. He was positive for the mutation, and his medical challenges came into sharp focus.

In 1990, when he was a baby, he was diagnosed with a massive brain tumor—an astrocytoma that originated near his thalamus, very close to his pituitary gland—that extended into his optic chiasm. When he was first diagnosed, I thought it was my fault. Even though I had no basis to think it was something genetic at the time, I had a pituitary tumor, so it seemed logical that I passed something on to him that caused him to have a tumor. Surgery, chemotherapy, and radiation eliminated his tumor, but there was a cost to becoming a childhood cancer survivor. The side effects of the treatment left him with life-long physical disabilities, partial blindness, and cognitive challenges. Being positive for the *AIP* mutation just seemed like too much of a coincidence not to be related. I was profoundly shaken by his results and overwhelmed with guilt that I caused him to have a life marred by his tumor that left him with so many disabilities.

When I asked Professor Korbonits if there was a correlation, she told me that the *AIP* gene mutation was not implicated in other types of tumors. However, if a sample of his tumor could be obtained, she would analyze it and decide if there was any connection. Finding a sample of his tumor seemed far-fetched, but I still had hope because my son's tumor biopsy was performed at Children's National Medical Center (CNMC) in Washington, DC, prior to his surgery in 1990. I told Professor Korbonits about the biopsy, thinking that there was no way that the sample could still exist and make its way to her in London. I should have known better than to underestimate her persistence.

Professor Korbonits tracked it down —it was preserved in paraffin wax and stored at CNMC—and persuaded them to send the sample to her. True to her word, a researcher in her laboratory analyzed it and gave me surprising results. My son's tumor was not caused by the mutation we shared. It was purely a coincidence.

As relief flooded over me, I realized that I learned a very valuable lesson about scientific research: correlation is not causation. In other words, just because two things occur at the same time does not mean they are related. Investigators must clearly understand cause and effect in their research without making invalid assumptions. Research conducted in labs like Professor Korbonits' demands rigorous testing and exacting research protocols to achieve valid results. Just because my son had a brain tumor did not mean that I was the cause, and having the *AIP* mutation did not make him immune to another type of tumor.

My questions initially focused on my immediate family. But what about my extended family? What about my sister? Both of her adult children had young children of their own. Were they at risk of inheriting a defective gene? Following the concept of cascade testing, it was time for my sister Cherie to be tested. Once again, obtaining the necessary justification for the DNA testing to satisfy the insurance company was a hassle, but she was able to get her testing done to see if she was a carrier. I knew that her height, 5 feet 2 inches, did not mean that she could not be a carrier, but it was still easy to assume that she was not one. The only way to know for sure is to take the test. I must admit I was surprised when her test came back positive. She was a carrier. Her two adult children were next up for testing. Her daughter was negative, while her son was positive, which meant his two children needed to be tested. We all were greatly relieved when they both came back negative. The testing showed that no descendants of my sister would ever have the genetic mutation.

Next, I looked at the other branches in my family tree. My mother had three brothers, all of whom could have inherited the mutation and passed it on to their children. I imagined each of my uncle's branches going out into the future. How many members of my extended family were at risk? What about my cousins on my mother's side? I was not close to my cousins: some I had only seen a few times as an adult, some I had never met. Two of my uncles were still alive, so I called them up to see if they would do the testing.

One of my uncles declined testing, so I contacted his son who also did not want to take the test because none of his children had children, so he didn't think it was important to take the test. I contacted my second uncle. He was willing to take the test, and fortunately it came back negative. That left my third uncle who died in 2015 in Colorado. I contacted his son and tried to persuade him and his siblings to get the testing done, but once again I hit a brick wall. Despite several emails and a phone call, they did not follow through.

I have puzzled over the reaction and the lack of interest in getting the testing done. I have seen first-hand how devastating the disease of gigantism can be and know the power of cascade testing, so it was hard for me to understand why someone would not take part in cascade testing when their family is at risk. I think there are three reasons. One, I think our healthcare system is a huge deterrent to the preventative care offered by cascade testing. When I talked with any of my relatives, the first question they asked me was how much the DNA test and doctor visits cost to get the testing done. I could not give them a straight answer. There was no way to tell exactly how much it would cost and precisely how they should go about getting the testing done. Two, they had never seen up-close the effects of gigantism. It was not a part of their life. They had never met me or knew anything about my medical history until I called them out of the blue, so they had no basis to understand the disease except for the dry, clinical information that I sent them. Three, I think that because the disease is so rare, and they had never heard of it, they were very leery to get involved with something that was difficult to understand. They could not see the value of knowing if they were a carrier. It just did not feel real enough to them to go through the hassle of getting the testing done.

The Holland family, on the other hand, experienced the positive benefits of cascade testing. It revealed family members at risk and led to effective treatment for Laura. In fact, in 2020, Professor Korbonits documented the benefits in one of her research papers "Significant Benefits of *AIP* Testing and Clinical Screening in Familial Isolated and Young-onset Pituitary Tumors," which was published in *The Journal of Clinical Endocrinology & Metabolism*.[1] The 12-year study determined that patients identified through cascade testing or population screening and followed through medical monitoring for symptoms of a pituitary tumor did better than patients who come into a clinical setting due to experiencing symptoms of a tumor. The study showed that the patients had smaller tumors with less brain damage. They also needed less treatment and fewer operations. The researchers recommended "germline *AIP* mutation genetic testing be offered at the earliest opportunity to first-degree relatives including children, because the disease may manifest by the age of 4."

Professor Korbonits emphasized how important it is to find the children who are carriers in a family that has the *AIP* mutation in their

_____

1  Pedro Marques et al., "Significant Benefits of *AIP* Testing and Clinical Screening in Familial Isolated and Young-onset Pituitary Tumors," *Journal of Clinical Endocrinology & Metabolism* 105, no. 6 (2020): e2247–60.

pedigree. The clinical benefits of early detection and monitoring are undeniable. "So, it could be totally devastating to be a giant. I mean, patients are
very wary that they are looked at on the street. There are data showing
that they are teased at school. It's something which is really horrible. So,
it's very important from a psychological point of view to avoid this as well.
But also, from the medical point of view, there are a lot of complications,
such as on the heart, on the bones, on the soft tissues, on their bowels, on
their jaw, really any part of their body." Diagnosing patients with a pituitary tumor is difficult with symptoms that span many medical special-
ties including neurology, cardiology, ophthalmology, orthopedics, and
dentistry, making it even more difficult to detect an undiagnosed tumor
before it can devastate someone's life. Cascade genetic testing holds the
very real possibility of changing the trajectory of lives and preventing a
genetic disease for generations to come.

# CHAPTER 8

# WE LIVE IN THE
# SHADOW OF EACH OTHER

**M**ore than a decade passed since Professor Korbonits and her team published their findings about the Northern Ireland *AIP* variant and its propensity to trigger a pituitary tumor before I made the connection between her research and my own pituitary tumor and found out I had the *AIP* mutation. My immediate reaction was relief. I now had the answer to my most pressing question: "why me?" The answer was clear: a genetic mutation caused my pituitary tumor. I also had the fascinating story of Charles Byrne to add to my family history. I must admit that having a literal skeleton in my family closet gave me a certain dark thrill.

While Brendan shared the same questions that I had about the direct impact on our families, his concerns were much broader than mine, reflecting his place in the community beyond his family. Right away, he could see the ramifications not only for his immediate family but also for his friends and neighbors.

When he thought about living in the geographic hotspot for the gene mutation, he thought about everyone he knew through his local historical society and Gaelic Athletic Association. His experience of being a modern-day giant in an area with giant-related landmarks and stories that tell tales of giants who have lived there for centuries encompassed his entire life. He was a living repository for giant-related information and helped others with acromegaly or gigantism find medical care. He knew intuitively that it was crucial to examine not only his family for the genetic anomaly but also his entire local community.

Like Brendan, Professor Korbonits and her team of endocrinologists were already thinking beyond their initial findings. It is important to make new discoveries, but even more important to discover how that research helps the patients. A population screening to determine the prevalence, or proportion of members in the total community who carry the defective gene, would provide valuable public health information. It promised to make the community aware of the disease, reveal undiagnosed cases of acromegaly and gigantism, and offer hope of preventing the deleterious effects of gigantism in the future. It would answer these basic questions. How prevalent is the gene variant in the population of this small area? How does the prevalence affect the local population? What recommendations can be made about screening in the future?

Brendan explained, "As time went on, it became clear that Professor Korbonits and her team proved beyond doubt that the *AIP* mutation was responsible for the high number of giants in south Derry and east Tyrone. A discussion arose as to what the exact prevalence of this gene in the area might be." When Brendan found out that Professor Korbonits obtained funding for a population genetic screening project in his community, he jumped right in and volunteered his time, energy, and connections to help the project. He pledged his full commitment to finding out the prevalence of the mutation near his home in Dungannon, in the heart of the geographic hotspot. First, they needed to come up with a plan to obtain the necessary DNA samples efficiently and effectively from community members.

As Professor Korbonits prepared the protocol for setting up the population screening and processing the DNA samples, Brendan turned his thoughts to the logistics of obtaining the samples. Brendan noted, "At the beginning, we thought we could achieve this with the assistance of local GP surgeries [general practitioner offices] in the area but that, on reflection, would have been very time consuming and expensive, as Professor Korbonits and her team would probably need to spend at least two weeks in the area. The funding for a project of that magnitude would have been out of the question, so we had to think more creatively."

Brendan reached out to Ronan who also knew the area. They brainstormed about alternate venues and came up with the idea of setting up in the parking lot of the local Tesco supermarkets. "Ronan's documentary had local impact, and it became quite popular in the community. Ronan was also very tied in with the local press," Brendan said. With Ronan's media contacts and Brendan's local ones, they began a campaign of raising awareness of the population screening in hopes of getting as much exposure as possible on television, radio, and in newspapers. They agreed that this plan would get the community interested, promote community involvement, and most importantly, lead to community members providing the necessary DNA samples.

After Brendan secured the agreement of the Tesco supermarkets for the population screening in Cookstown on February 8 and 9 and Dungannon on March 1 and 2, 2013, Brendan set off on a media blitz with Professor Korbonits available to provide her medical expertise when needed. The BBC Northern Ireland radio flagship news program, *Good Morning Ulster* invited them to appear, and local newspapers including the Dungannon-based *Tyrone Times*, the Cookstown-based *Mid Ulster Herald,* and the Omagh-based *Ulster Herald* went a long way to getting the word out about the project. RTÉ Radio Dublin picked up the story and interviewed Brendan and Niamh on a popular afternoon program. The campaign gathered momentum when the University of London's publicity department joined in to help reach the UK audience.

Brendan also credits his Gaelic Athletic Association (GAA) connections with helping garner interest in the project. Since its founding in 1884, the GAA has been an important sport and cultural institution in Ireland, promoting not only traditional Irish sports, such as hurling and Gaelic football, but also Irish language, music, and dance. "The GAA contributes greatly to our sense of community. Every family has someone involved in the GAA. You form relationships with other members that makes you very aware of and responsible to the community. It's a big part of how we think and live. Sport for us is very much about public health. There's an Irish saying: We all live in the shadow of each other. We feel a great responsibility to those we share the same piece of earth with."

He told me about a man that he met at a Gaelic football game. "A mutual friend introduced me to Tony Guerin, and I immediately recognized that he was suffering from acromegaly. He had a protruding brow and jawbone, thickened skin, enlarged fingers, and wide feet so characteristic of the condition. After some small talk, I asked him if he suffered from headaches. He gave me a quizzical look and after a pause admitted he did have very severe headaches. I told him he should consult his doctor at once as he might have this rare medical condition. Later, I learned from my friend that this man was a Special Branch detective in Dublin. He asked our mutual friend if I was some sort of quack. My friend explained that I was deadly serious, and that he should take my advice to heart. Apparently, he did contact his doctor and was properly diagnosed and treated. He called later to thank me and to tell me that he had his first night of full sleep in 20 years."

As the day for the population screening neared, Brendan, with the help of his son Michael, completed his share of the planning for the testing. Michael set up portable offices in the Tesco parking lots, while Brendan recruited community volunteers and organized meals and accommodations for the endocrinologists, geneticists, and other researchers staying locally over the two weekends while conducting the screening. Brendan relied on his community connections to help. "I am one of the founders of the Killeeshil & Clonaneese Historical Society, so I asked our members to help. One of our officers, Jonathan Gray, provided valuable assistance. I was also able to get locally cooked meals and take excellent care of the researchers while they were here." The logistics were in place for the population screening.

Professor Korbonits obtained ethical permission to conduct the public screening and assembled her team of researchers from the United Kingdom, Bangladesh, Italy, Mexico, Czech Republic, Hungary, and Romania. Over the course of two weekends, they hoped to amass enough DNA samples to answer their key questions.

Researchers Dr. Serbian Radian and Dr. Maria Herincs commented on their hope for a successful screening. "Realising that this part of the world is very special in terms of the genetics of pituitary tumours, we decided to go on a genetic epidemiology 'expedition' to two small Northern Irish towns....Giving up 10 minutes of time and providing personal details as well as a 2 ml of saliva for DNA extraction, may not seem like much, but it is probably not what most of us have in mind when we rush out for our shopping at the local supermarket!"[1]

Excitement grew as Brendan went to greet the medical team at Belfast International Airport when they arrived from London. "While the team of young researchers in endocrinology came from very different and varying countries and cultures, it became apparent very quickly that they were very focused and committed to seeing the project through to a successful conclusion." All the pieces were now in place for the population screening to begin the next day even though no one knew if anyone would show up for the testing.

The bright blue t-shirts with the slogan "Endocrinologists do it with Hormones" set the tone for the day despite the overcast skies and cool misty rain.

Located in the large gray portable offices in the parking lot, the researchers organized their stacks of consent forms and lined up plastic

---

1 Serban Radian and Maria Herincs, "Legends and Facts: Population Screening for AIP Mutations in Northern Ireland," *The Endocrinologist*, Summer 2013, 24.

vials to collect the needed saliva for the DNA testing. After filling the vial with 2 ml of saliva from study participants, the lids would be clicked into place and filed for later processing. As the scientists snapped on their latex gloves, they were hopeful that many community members would take advantage of the testing. Placards with information about the pituitary gland and pituitary disorders and images of famous Irish giants hung on the doors and windows of the makeshift office. Additional posters with details about the intriguing story of Charles Byrne and the legacy of gigantism in the area were set up on easels inside the Tesco supermarkets.

Bustling with excitement as they opened the doors to the portable offices at 7 am, the endocrinologists set to work as community members began arriving, despite the early hour. It quickly became clear that the screening was a success, much to the delight of the researchers and the community volunteers. Michael, Brendan's son, pointed out how willing people were to join in. "My overall role was mostly getting infrastructure in place, but I was there that day, and it was very noticeable that a lot of people saw the news reports and said, hey I better get tested, that seems a noteworthy thing to do. So, there wasn't a lot of goading anyone to do the test. They came of their own accord."

Brendan recruited his brother Aidan to help with the effort. Aidan remembered how exciting the day was as more and more people responded to efforts to get tested for the benefit of the community. He told them about the process and encouraged them to participate. "We had to explain to anybody who gave a saliva sample what the project was about. We went up to them and asked them if they wanted to take part and most people didn't mind doing it. They didn't know anything about gigantism but once you explained what it was that you were trying to do, they got behind the idea. There was only one odd crank who complained, and I was the one to find him. But mostly once you explained the procedure, everybody was quite willing to give a sample."

Julian Fowler, reporter with BBC News Northern Ireland, interviewed researchers, volunteers, and screening participants on the first weekend. He spoke with Professor Patrick Morrison, clinical geneticist at Belfast City Hospital, who linked the project to the legend of Fionn Mac Cumhaill and modern-day gigantism. "We think [this area] may be one of the cradles of giant civilization. We don't know if Fionn Mac Cumhaill started here and headed up to the north coast but certainly we've one or two people who we've identified here who are certainly 6 foot 9 and 6 foot 10, so certainly quite a few giants around."[2] Fowler emphasized the importance of the genetic discovery to the families in east Tyrone and south Derry and encouraged their participation.

Fowler also spoke with Professor Korbonits about why the research is so valuable to the local community. She pointed out that in addition to the testing, the team also took the opportunity to write to local doctors to tell them about the screening and educate them about the prevalence of the disease in the area. "[We know] that over two-thirds of those who carry the mutation do not develop the condition, and therefore, they have no idea that they carry the gene abnormality."

Fowler's reporting bolstered interest as more and more people arrived in the parking lot throughout the day and into the next. As the day ended, the researchers noted that they collected samples for 12 hours at a rate of about 19 samples per hour. They continued this pace for the remaining days of the population screening. As Drs. Radian and Herincs pointed out, "With the ideal mixture of determination, resourcefulness and skill from all those involved, but most of all with the generosity of the volunteers taking part in the study, the team managed to collect an impressive 956 saliva samples in 48 hours."[3] The community

---

2 Julian Fowler, "Land of the Giants?," *BBC News*, February 8, 2013, https://www.bbc.com/news/av/uk-northern-ireland-21387358.

3 Serban Radian and Maria Herincs, "Legends and Facts: Population Screening for AIP Mutations in Northern Ireland," *The Endocrinologist*, Summer 2013, 24.

response was far greater than anticipated. The population screening was a resounding success.

When Brendan first told me about this research, I was astonished that close to 1000 people were willing to give a sample of their DNA in the parking lot of the local Tesco. It was very hard for me to imagine a similar setup in a Walmart parking lot near my Virginia home, a conservative stronghold in a rural community. If done in the US, I anticipated the skepticism that would arise from an appeal to donate DNA for a research project. I thought that people would be very leery of undergoing DNA testing and distrustful of how the data from the testing would be used. During the pandemic, the value of public health measures was hotly debated, and the idea of simply doing something for the common good of the community was called into question. I could imagine questions about whether researchers stood to gain financially from obtaining the DNA or if the data derived from the study would be used outside the scope of the stated intent. Why were people in the Tesco parking lots so willing to give their DNA to the researchers?

When I posed this question to Michael, Brendan's son, he responded by referring to the differences in our healthcare systems. The National Health Service (NHS) is a unified system that is publicly funded and community-based, while the American system is a fragmented mixture of for-profit insurers, private health provider businesses, and government run programs without a direct public health, community-based component. "People here don't look at medical care as a business. It's not a business; it's a service that you pay for through your taxes. The National Health Service 99% of the time gets it right, the rest is human error. There's a trust there. Unlike with the private health care companies in the States, you don't have the angle of anyone making money. You don't wonder about some ulterior thought behind it. We have a sense of public health. Most people here are of the opinion that if you can help somebody out by giving them whatever they need, it will come back to you down the road. It's basically karma."

The researchers were delighted with the turnout and the samples collected, but the scope and importance of the population screening went beyond the DNA data collected. Many of the participants told stories about giants known in the local community. Some brought photographs or newspaper clippings of relatives they suspected had gigantism. For example, Dr. Cecilia Ward, a retired local pediatrician, showed the scientists a clipping from a newspaper published in May 1913 in Canada titled, "Ireland Loses Her Tallest Boy," featuring her 21-year-old uncle upon his arrival in Canada. At 6 feet, 10 inches (208 cm), he stood more than a head taller than the men around him, and his elongated face and large feet mark him as having gigantism. Sadly, he died less than a month later from a hypertensive crisis, a known complication of gigantism. While intriguing, the story of her uncle was not the only tale she wanted to share.

Because she was aware of gigantism in her own family, Dr. Ward saved an article in the west Donegal publication *The Rosses Annual* about the discovery of a giant skeleton in February 1954 on Cruit Island on Donegal's west coast. Local workers, while digging gravel for road repairs, unearthed human bones a mere eight inches below the surface. Lying on his back in a burlap sack, the remains appeared to be a huge man with long hair and a full set of teeth. His position suggested that he was deliberately buried, along with a small collection of coins, among the shifting sands of the tiny island overlooking a sheltered inlet.

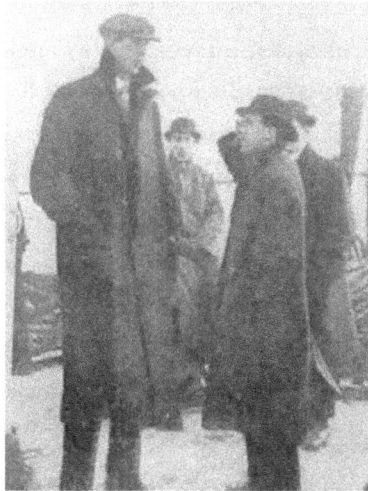

"Ireland Loses Her Tallest Boy"

The article noted that local coroner Dr. McGinley examined the remains. He believed the man died in early adolescence, and that he suffered from pituitary gigantism. After the examination, the giant skeleton was reinterred on the island in Cill Bhride cemetery, a short distance from where he was found. Although the newspaper article noted the burial, the exact location of his bones within the cemetery is still unknown.

Stories like the ones told by Dr. Ward offered valuable clues to past cases of gigantism in the community. Even more crucially, the screening addressed concerns that participants had about themselves or living family members. Brendan remembered one incident. "We were visited by the parents of very tall children. The medical team directed them to seek medical advice, possibly leading to early intervention and treatment. If one child was identified and diagnosed, then all the work the team had undertaken would be worth it. In one case I met a young man who seemed to me to have all the outward symptoms of a pituitary tumor. When I met him, it was like reliving my youth or looking in a mirror, seeing my reflection from forty years ago."

Aidan, Brendan's brother, recalled meeting one mother who expressed concern about her son. "One woman I was speaking to said that her son, who was still a teenager, was much taller than average. I told her to go and have a word with [Professor Korbonits] and they arranged to bring the lad in that evening. It was very satisfying that she was giving us her professional knowledge. That was probably one of the most important things that came out of the screening."

The population screening was a decisive success, but the researchers' work was far from finished. They needed to analyze the DNA samples. This would allow them to show whether the region they identified as a geographic hotspot indeed had a significantly higher prevalence of the gene that caused gigantism in the general population. Figuring out the prevalence of the specific Northern Ireland *AIP* mutation in contrast to another area in Ireland would give them the answer. After returning to London, Professor Korbonits' team obtained genetic information from patients who participated previously in the Greater Belfast PRIME study and the Republic of Ireland (ROI) Trinity Biobank. They obtained 1000

DNA profiles from the Belfast study and 2,094 from the Trinity Biobank to create two large control groups. It took three years to complete their comparative analysis and arrive at their conclusions.

Their findings and recommendations were published in 2017 in the journal *Human Mutation* under the title "Increased Population Risk of *AIP*-Related Acromegaly and Gigantism in Ireland."[4] The publication recognized forty-eight authors, including Brendan, his brother Aidan, and Ronan, in acknowledgement of their substantial contributions to the research project. The researchers found that the population screening revealed several subjects with the Northern Ireland variant, confirming the area identified as a geographic hotspot. The data suggested that the mutation is present in the area, justifying vigilance for rapidly growing teenagers and testing for all young patients with acromegaly or prolactinoma who are from the area. This stood in stark contrast to the data from the Trinity Biobank which had zero cases of the *AIP* variant. The Greater Belfast PRIME study had only one positive sample.

Undeniably, the Northern Ireland community west of Lough Neagh benefited from the population screening and the valuable medical insights derived from the findings in the research paper. Likewise, the researchers who came to the two Irish towns to gather data also came away from the experience changed. They left their laboratories to go out to the test site, engage with community members, hear their concerns about their children, and come face-to-face with patients affected by the disease of gigantism and acromegaly. Instead of sterile facts and laboratory specimens, they met flesh and blood patients directly affected by gigantism.

Before returning to their home countries, the research team went with Brendan on a field trip to Littlebridge on the eastern fringes of the Sperrin Mountains, where Charles Byrne once made his home in the late 1700s.

---

4 Harvinder S. Radian et al., "Increased Population Risk of *AIP*-Related Acromegaly and Gigantism in Ireland," *Human Mutation* 38, no. 1 (2017): 78-85.

As they gathered for a group photograph, Brendan thanked the international team. He commended them not only for their professional expertise but also for their remarkable enthusiasm and intense interest in the local community, which was affected by the *AIP* mutation. The story of Charles Byrne is compelling, yet ghoulish in the details of how his skeleton came to hang in the Hunterian Museum in London. But his story didn't end there. It circles back to his native homeland through the scientific exploration of the genetic legacy that gave him his gigantism and continues to affect the lives of the local community. While his bones may be in London, his soul surely remains in Northern Ireland among the scenic beauty of Littlebridge and the enduring genetic heritage of his birthplace.

# CHAPTER 9

# THE LAND OF GIANTS

Two years had ticked by since I first met Brendan, and by January 2022 I could feel the pressure of the pandemic lifting ever so slightly as vaccines became more readily available, the anti-viral pill Paxlovid came on to the market, the mask mandate was lifted, and quarantine time dropped to five days. The death toll climbed past 800,000 and the new Covid strains Delta and Omicron frayed nerves, but there was hope that we might be able to get to the other side and have normal lives again when travel restrictions eased. The door to the world cracked open, and I was ecstatic when my sister and I started planning our trip to Northern Ireland for May.

For the last two years, I was immersed in a virtual world of giants, and now was my chance to meet Brendan in the flesh and see for myself the land of the giants I read about online. With my sister Cherie in Arkansas and me in Virginia, our plan was to meet at London's Heathrow Airport and then fly to Belfast together. I welcomed her company. Having lived in England 20 years ago, she knew how to drive on the left-hand side of the road. She became the driver for our adventure.

Like many Americans, before I found out that my ancestors were from Northern Ireland not from what is now the Republic of Ireland, I didn't fully understand that the island of Ireland is divided into two political entities: the twenty-six counties of the Republic of Ireland with Dublin as its capital and the six counties of Northern Ireland, which is part of the United Kingdom, with Belfast as its capital. Traveling to Northern Ireland meant that I was leaving behind the stereotypical images of shamrocks and leprechauns tinged with emerald green found in the south that most Americans associate with Ireland. I was heading north to what was once the ancient kingdom of Ulster, a region with its own distinct history and imagery.

When we landed at George Best Belfast City Airport, that imagery came into sharp focus. The bold red hand of Ulster replaced the green shamrocks that symbolize the Republic of Ireland to the south. Spectacular over-sized photographs of the rugged Antrim coastline, the massive walls of Derry, and the dramatic beauty of the Sperrin Mountains in County Tyrone lined the passageways through the airport. Tourism Northern Ireland's slogan "Embrace a Giant Spirit" framed each of the pictures. Unlike the leprechauns of the south, there was nothing diminutive in the imagery associated with Northern Ireland.

We lingered in Belfast for a few days to enjoy the gritty industrial vibe of a city that was once a shipbuilding titan that created the ill-fated ship the Titanic. We visited the Peace Walls and learned how Belfast survived the Troubles, and we savored the city's excellent eateries and pubs. But I was eager to head north. I wanted to meet the ancient giants of Northern Ireland found at the Giant's Causeway on the Antrim coast.

The dense urban neighborhoods of northern Belfast quickly gave way to rolling countryside as we headed to the north coast. After the sensory deprivation of the pandemic, I could feel the world around me pop with color as we drove along. I fell in love with the spring green meadows surrounded by bright yellow gorse hedgerows that marked the fields dotted with Blackface Mountain sheep and Holstein dairy cows. Cherie pointed out the farmhouses as they came into view, many atop the hillocks that overlooked the pastoral beauty. We drove to the far north where the road ended at the sea and parked at the Causeway Hotel, perched on the top of the Aird Snout cliffs. I breathed in the smell of the salty brine that filled the air as we gazed out onto the water. We both relished the views across the Atlantic Ocean from the promontory. They were dramatic with the town of Portrush clinging to the coastline to the west and Rathlin Island to the east with its own impressive cliffs and array of birds and wildflowers.

While the scene from on top of the cliffs was breathtaking, it was the rocks that we came to see. As my sister and I descended on the pathway that wound its way down to the shoreline from the cliffs, I was awe-struck by the commanding presence of the rock pillars that formed the base of the cliffs. Waves crashed against the coastline, eddying between the dramatic hexagonal stones that jutted out into the Atlantic Ocean. More than 40,000 of the interlocking hexagonal columns of basalt followed along the shoreline for four plus miles. The columns varied in height from just a foot or two to towering over us more than forty feet high. Unusual stone groupings and shapes with fanciful names such as the Giant's Boot spread across the shoreline. Giant's Eyes, water pools in depressions on top of the columns, dotted the rock formations.

I watched as the kittiwake gulls screeched and swooped across the dynamic landscape, diving down from the cliffs. The distinctive stones of the Giant's Causeway appeared to reach out across the water to Scotland's Island of Staffa only thirty miles away. It was easy to see why the site has thrilled visitors to Ireland's northern coast long before its designation as a UNESCO World Heritage Site in 1986. I was awed by the stones' majesty and understood why ancient people gazed up in wonder at the majestic rocks as they tried to understand how the unusual columns came into being.

Scientists say that the rocks were formed sixty million years ago when molten lava rapidly cooled, fracturing into the distinctive columnar shape of the rocky formation. Science says that volcanic activity forged the geological wonder, but ancient stories tell a different tale.

According to local lore a mythological giant created the distinctive landscape when Fionn Mac Cumhaill (often anglicized to Finn MacCool) leader of the elite Fenian warriors bent the local landscape to his will. Stories of the feats of Mac Cumhaill abound. One story tells of when in a fit of rage as he prepared for battle, Fionn tore a clump of earth from the ground and hurled it into the Irish Sea, creating the Isle of Mann with Lough Neagh, Ireland's largest freshwater lake, forming in the void left behind.

Another story tells of how the Giant's Causeway came into being when the Scottish giant Benandonner challenged Fionn to a fight. Fionn created the columnar pathway to connect Ireland and Scotland and gain access to his enemy. Some stories say that Fionn defeated Benandonner easily and then ripped up the stones that stretched to Scotland to keep Benandonner from returning. Other stories tell a more complicated tale of trickery with Fionn's wife Oonagh playing a prominent role in deceiving the Scottish giant who fled in terror at the very thought of fighting Fionn. While the tales may differ what is undeniable is that they show off the colossal power of Fionn to alter the landscape through his sheer physical presence and strength. He is both powerful and creative, a force of nature standing tall against the crashing waves at the Causeway.

As I looked out on to the sea and then back to the towering rock formation behind me with the sun beaming down and the chill wind in my face, I knew I was in the land of the giants—a land so beautiful that Fionn Mac Cumhaill stood ready to guard its beauty with his life.

Like modern day scientists who observe natural phenomenon and seek to understand why certain marvels exist, ancient people sought to understand the world around them. As I looked out on the otherworldly beauty of the Giant's Causeway, I understood why legends develop. Humans seek patterns. We seek explanations for what appears inexplicable. We want to satisfy our curiosity. When we see an anomaly, we want to understand. Mythology offers a path of imagination to explain the unusual. Legends fill the gap between the known and unknown by imagining how something of such beauty could exist. Through imagination, we can embrace the world with all its anomalies with awe and wonder.

Cherie and I stopped off at the Causeway Hotel's Parlour restaurant for a beer before continuing our journey by winding our way west along the coastline to spend the afternoon at Portstewart Strand. As I sipped on my Inish Mac Saint IPA, with its label depicting Fionn Mac Cumhaill, I filled my sister in on some of the other landmarks in Northern Ireland with place-names linked to giants that Brendan told me about during one of our many video meetings. As a local historian, Brendan had a particular interest in landmarks and place-names that pointed to real people, real giants who may have inhabited the land around him. For him, these names showed just how deeply giant lore is ingrained into the very topography of Northern Ireland, especially in Counties Tyrone and Derry. Brendan told me that if I wanted proof of giants living in Northern Ireland, I should consult the Northern Ireland Place-Name Project.

When I looked up the project, I was amazed at how extensive it was and the level of detail provided online. Developed by the Department of Irish & Celtic Studies at Queen's University, Belfast, the project's database (www.placenamesni.org) has the origins and meanings of over 30,000 place-names in Northern Ireland. The database offers tantalizing clues to locations where giants might have lived through place-names with a link to giants. When I put "giant" into the database search bar, fifty-eight locations referencing giants came up. Some place-names were solely descriptive, such as the Giant's Ring, but what jumped out at me was how forty-one of them were listed as a giant's grave. Twenty-two of those graves clustered in a tight geographic area near Cookstown in County Tyrone.

My sister laughed at me when I told her how this one database search result set me off on a whole afternoon of googling place-names. She knew me well enough to know how much I loved rabbit holes when I am researching so she wasn't surprised when I mentioned that I went off on a deep dive, barely coming up for air when the importance of place-names in Ireland grabbed my interest. I told her that I discovered just how valued place-names are in Ireland when I came across the Tailte Éireann, an entire government agency dedicated to maintaining the historical records of mapping and surveying of landmarks throughout the island of Ireland not just in the north. A blog post by Risteard Ua Cróinín, Architectural Conservation Officer and Archaeologist for the Clare County Council summed up the importance when he wrote, "Where no written record remains of past civilisation or the day-to-day events of ordinary people, much remains to be unlocked from information contained in the names of townlands, streets, rivers, fields and monuments."[1]

After we paid our bill, headed back to the car, and set off for Portstewart, I couldn't resist telling her the story of a giant's grave in County Tyrone and how it is related to the classic 18th century book *Gulliver's Travels*. Most people are familiar with the book by Anglo-Irish storyteller and satirist Jonathan Swift, which features the giant Lemuel Gulliver who towers over the Lilliputians. The book also features a race of giants known as the Brobdingnagians who likewise dwarf Gulliver. Swift was close friends with a man named Robert Lindesay, who often hosted Swift between 1720 and 1725 at his home Loughry Manor on his estate in County Tyrone. Swift penned much of *Gulliver's Travels*, while staying in a small cottage next to Lindesay's home.

During my research into place-names, I discovered the online National Irish Library and when I delved into its vast online holdings, I came across an intriguing circa-1901 sketchbook that contained a drawing of a giant's grave located on Robert Lindesay's estate.[2] The drawing was a re-creation of a sketch from the early 1800s labeled Giant's Grave. The drawing depicted a 25 ft. x 7 ft. rectangle of ancient stones set in a grove of trees and oriented on an east/west axis. Two large rocks lie across the foot of the rectangle. The stone landmark can still be seen to this day.

---

1 Risteard Ua Cróinín, *Clare County Library*, www.clarelibrary.ie/eolas/coclare/places/importance_of_placenames.htm.

2 William Frazer and G. Henry (George Henry) Kinahan. Giant's Grave, Loughry Demesne, County Tyrone, National Library of Ireland, Sketch Books of Irish Antiquities. Catalogue No. PD 1975 TX 27 (29).

Swift must have known about the Giant's Grave referenced in Frazer's drawing. It is easy to imagine Swift visiting the Giant's Grave, hearing local tales of mythological giants, meeting someone with gigantism in the known geographic hotspot for the disease, and finding inspiration to weave his tale of Lemuel Gulliver in the land of the Lilliputians.

We followed the winding road that twisted and turned along the rugged granite bluffs with a sheer drop to the ocean, huge boulders at the foot of the crags, and pounding surf tossing salty water in the air. We passed the turn off for the seaside resort town of Portstewart, situated on a high cliff, and took a narrow road down to the beaches of the Portstewart Strand.

Dark gray clouds scuttled across the sky as the sun peeked through in luminescent streaks while we walked out on to the wide golden sandy beach. The waves lapped against the shoreline, at times reaching the small pools further inland that were filled with brown and white seashells. To our left, ancient sand dunes sheltered curlew and redshank birds among its thickets of hawthorn trees and elder shrubs. As I walked along, my feet sinking into the wet sand, I could see my sister bending, looking intently for shells, a familiar sight from our many beach trips to the Atlantic beaches in the US. I stopped and realized I was on the other side of the same ocean that I have loved for as long as I can remember. The sea, the sky, and the sand welcomed me, and I was at peace in this land as I imagined fellow giants finding a comfortable home here as well among the sweeping vistas, the golden sands, and grandeur of the ocean before me.

We spent the night near Bushmill on the north coast, and I woke up energized and itching to get on the road. The plan was to meet Brendan at a church near Coalisland where some of my ancestors were buried. Brendan pulled together a tour through the countryside to see many of the places that we talked about over the past two years and arranged for Julian Fowler of BBC Northern Ireland to interview us about how we met. I was excited to get there, but I was equally enthusiastic about what we would see on the way.

Cherie and I decided to drive south through the Sperrin Mountains, a sparsely populated 40-mile mountain range of boglands and heather-covered hills along the border of counties Tyrone and Derry. Over the past year, I started to study the Irish language, which unlocked another layer for me to explore in my research about the giant legends and folklore of Northern Ireland when I came across stories written in Irish. Now I had the chance to see the land of giants described in that giant folklore.

One book stood out for me: *Sgéalta Mhuintir Luinigh: Munterloney Folktales: Irish Traditions from County Tyrone* by folklorist Eámonn Ó Tuathails. Ó Tuathails traveled through the Munterloney area in the center of the Sperrins in 1933 to gather stories and poetry from traditional storytellers who lived there. The stories portray a land filled with magical creatures—sprites, fairies, Little People, and witches—that beguile the humans while giants loom over the landscape, shaping the very contours of the land.

I met up once again with Fionn Mac Cumhaill in some of these folktales, as he throws stones to show off his might and beat back other giants who threaten to invade. However, not all giants I read about in the *Munterloney Folktales* are larger than life and powerful. I was fascinated by how the giants were depicted in the story "*Na Trí Fathach*/The Three Giants."[3] It is a tale of three brothers who lived in the mountains and "fatnach a bhí ina ngach a'n duine acu" which translates as "giant was in each of them." The translation caught my interest because it made me think about how a genetic mutation is intrinsic to a person with gigantism.

The story goes that the giants were enormously wealthy, yet physically flawed, each with only one eye on their forehead. At a local dance, a young boy boasts that he can make off with the giants' hoard of gold and silver. The other fellows bet him a thousand pounds that he can't. The

3  Eámonn Ó Tuathail, *Sgéalta Mhuintir Luinigh: Munterloney Folktales: Irish Traditions from County Tyrone* (The Folklore of Ireland Council, 193; reprint 2015), 67-69.

boy takes the challenge and rides off to meet the giants. He stops at each of the giants' houses, easily duping them into believing that he is there to save them from robbers who are on their way to kill them. The boy tricks them into giving him their treasure in exchange for his protection. He locks them up to hide them from the would-be robbers and takes off with the giants' treasure, returning triumphant to the dance to collect on his bet. The giants' size does not save them. They are weak and ineffectual, believing a young boy needs to protect them.

There was another story in the book that I loved because I felt like I was reading about a real person who once lived in the Sperrin Mountains. "An Fathach ÓCléirigh/Giant O'Clery"[4] is a magical tale of the Little People, mischievous sprites eager to spirit off children, waiting outside the window of a woman in childbirth. They peer into the window riveted on the midwife, waiting for her to place the child in the cradle, a moment when they can reach in and snatch the unbaptized child away. Fortunately, O'Clery sees them gathering by the window and starts towards the house. When the Little People see him, they scurry off in fear. The giant takes note of their departure but lingers through the night to guard the inhabitants. He is a protective force that ensures the baby's safety until morning when the child will be baptized and no longer threatened by the Little People. I was struck by how powerful yet ordinary O'Clery is portrayed in the story. He is a valued member of the community, offering security and comfort.

One other online resource stood out for me when I was doing my folklore research: the National Folklore Collection UCD Digitization Project's The Schools' Collection.[5] From 1937 to 1939, thousands of schoolchildren and their teachers from schools in the twenty-six counties of Ireland collected folktales, legends, proverbs, poems, and oral history from their parents, grandparents, and neighbors. While the project didn't

4 Ibid., 259-260.

5 National Folklore Collection, UCD, "The Schools' Collection," 2023, duchas.ie, www.duchas.ie/en/cbes.

cover the six counties of Northern Ireland, some stories were from County Donegal which borders Counties Tyrone and Derry.

When I read the poem "The Gray Stone on the Heath" by James Mc Loughlin recorded by teacher Donnachadh E. Mac Congáile, I could feel the humanity of the giant shepherd depicted in the poem. The poem starts with a description of a local stone landmark known as the Giant's Seat just west of the Sperrin Mountains in the Finn Valley near the town of Killygordon. The poet contemplates the huge gray boulder shaped like a chair and imagines it as a relic of a giant race "that ruled ere Fionn held sway," but then he thinks of another option—a quite human option—a giant shepherd. The giant shepherd is a man of the land, tending his sheep while gazing across the valley as he rests on his giant stone chair. It was easy for me to imagine this giant as we rolled through the countryside with hills dotted with sheep.

As we neared Coalisland, we realized our time was short to get to the church for our meeting with Brendan and Julian, so we needed to cut out one stop that I really wanted to make because of its connection to giant folklore. The Beaghmore Stones are one of many stone circles found throughout Ireland dating back to the Bronze Age. They are a complex array of stone circles and cairns aligned astronomically with the phases of the moon and the summer solstice. The giant mythology behind these stones is what captivated me and roots them in the giant folklore tradition of the Sperrins.

Legend has it that when night falls on the summer solstice, the large stones transform into giants who dance throughout the darkness until first light comes when the giants solidify back into stones to wait until the next solstice's sunset when they can rise again in celebration. As we passed the turn off for the Beaghmore Stones, I promised myself that one day I'd return to see them.

When we turned on to Mountjoy Rd. for the final few miles of our day's journey, I wondered what it was going to be like to meet Brendan physically. We developed a firm friendship based not only on our shared gigantism but also our interests in Irish history and legends. He was the one that encouraged me to learn to speak Irish, which I found further tied me to my ancestral home. I already knew him, but it was mostly through a computer screen, flat and two-dimensional. I thought back to when I first saw him when I watched the documentary about Charles Byrne. I remembered Brendan's introductory scene.

The scene opens with Brendan walking up a country lane alone past light green hedgerows, with darkening clouds behind him, silhouetting his broad shoulders and towering frame. As he nears the camera his facial features come into focus. Although his face is fine-featured with a bit of boyishness despite being 60 years old in the film, I was still able to see the characteristics of someone marked by giantism or acromegaly in his prominent chin and brow. I also noticed how large his hands and feet appeared. When the camera zoomed in even closer and Brendan began to reflect on the difficult life of fellow giant Charles Byrne, I felt the warm compassion in Brendan's voice and the kindness in his eyes that I grew to appreciate as we got to know each other online.

I snapped back to the present when we rounded the corner and St. Michael's Church of Ireland came into view. We pulled into the gravel driveway of the simple church, known as the Clonoe Chapel by locals, situated on a slight rise in the green flatlands that extend to Lough Neagh. White lichens covered the gray stones of the quaint chapel which was surrounded by gravestones dating back to the 1700s. I heard the crunch of another car pulling up and saw Brendan in the passenger seat. I jumped out of the car but then hesitated, unsure of exactly how to greet him. A hug seemed presumptuous and a handshake way too formal. When he opened his door, any worries I had vanished when I saw his warm smile, and he became alive and three-dimensional right before my eyes. It was Brendan, my good friend, so of course a hug was the way to go.

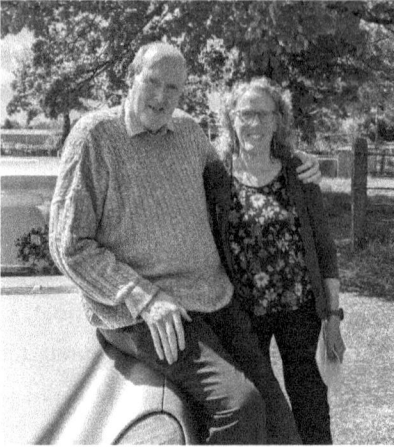

Brendan and Colleen

Brendan struggled to get out of the car, which took me aback. But then, I realized that the documentary, made ten years prior to our meeting, captured Brendan while he was still moving easily, and walking down the road posed no challenge. Over the intervening ten years, his body was worn down by the negative effects of his gigantism. His mobility was reduced, and he often used a wheelchair to get around. He developed heart disease, which further restricted his movement. He mentioned to me that it was hard for him to walk more than 50 yards.

I knew that he was deeply affected physically, but I also understood that he was not broken. His stature was not just in the height of his body; it was also in the expanse of his sympathetic spirit. He was an undeniable presence—a presence I noticed from the first moment I encountered him in the film and now saw in front of me for the first time. I reached up to hug him when he stood, and as he made his way to the front of the car to lean on the hood, I linked arms with him for a photograph that secured a moment I looked forward to for a long time.

We barely had time to talk before Julian arrived and set up his camera for our interview for the BBC.[6] Julian was already familiar with the overall story and Professor Korbonits' research because of his coverage of the population screening. Brendan and I perched on a low stone wall as we answered Julian's questions about how we met. I also explained to him why we opted to meet at the church.

---

6 Julian Fowler, "Acromegaly: 'Giant gene' bond forged between Us and Mid Ulster," *BBC Northern Ireland,* www.bbc.com/news/uk-northern-ireland-61726811, accessed October 29, 2023.

Before my trip, Brendan connected me with his close friend Rita Kelly McCaughey, a genealogist in Australia, in hopes of finding out more about my family's history in Ireland. A fire in 1922 at the Public Records Office of Ireland in Dublin during the Irish Civil War destroyed many documents such as census returns, legal records, and testamentary wills that genealogical researchers typically rely on for their information. Rita, however, consulted local parish records, which included birth, baptism, marriage, and death records to provide me with the needed information. Rita traced my history back to the 1740s and told me that two of my relatives, one who died in 1741 and the other in 1792, were buried in the graveyard of St. Michael's Church. Unfortunately, she couldn't tell me the exact location of the graves, so Julian filmed Cherie and me as we searched among the chiseled headstones, many with lettering obscured through weathering over the centuries. We didn't find the headstones that day, but I was happy to know that I was among my ancestors.

As we waved goodbye to Julian and started to get in our cars, I felt a renewed sense of excitement when I thought about our next stop: the site of the McGuirk tenancy. Before our trip, I found the location of the land using the information from Rita about where my ancestors once lived in Clonoe parish when Brendan suggested that I check the Griffith's Valuation property tax survey from 1847 to 1864 to see if I could find any Clonoe land records related to the John Robert McGuirk's father John McGuirk.[7]

When I plugged the information into the Griffith's Valuation search engine and clicked, one record came up for John McGuirk the elder, which listed him as living on plot 29 with a house and garden that measured

---

7  Conducted between 1847 and 1864, the Griffith's Valuation was a property tax survey that mapped all the landholdings in Ireland along with basic information about the property and the tenants who lived on the land. The Valuation has been digitized and is available online. The Valuation records were unaffected by the 1922 Dublin fire. The records are one of the most important 19th century sources for genealogical research and to understand the catastrophic effects of the Great Famine of 1845-48. www.askaboutireland. ie/griffith-valuation/index.xml

13 perches and a rateable annual valuation of one pound, five shillings.[8] Another click took me to the 19th-century Valuation map showing plot 29. To my amazement, the website also included a modern road map overlay showing exactly how to get to the land, which was roughly on the corner of Cloghog Rd. and Washingbay Rd., only two miles from the church where we stood. Brendan arranged for his friend James Walshe, a local storyteller with tales about local history and legends, to be our guide.

As we rolled through the countryside, I was struck once again by the incredible beauty of the land and couldn't help wondering how my great-great-great grandmother felt as she watched her eleven-year-old son set off for America, never to be seen again.

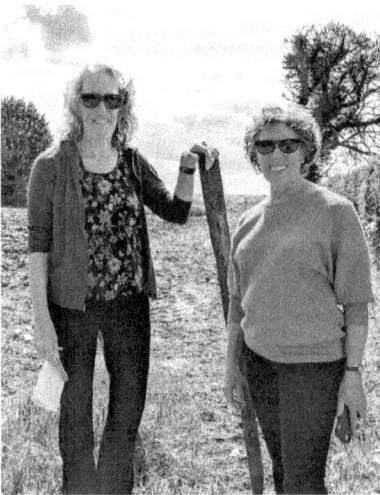

Cherie and Colleen at the McGuirk tenant farm

Suddenly, James told us to pull over on the side of the road near a rustic gate and pointed to a small field tilled into rows for potato planting. Blue skies shone through puffy white clouds as I stood looking out on the tiny plot of land. After first seeing the description of the land in Griffith's Valuation, I did the math to figure out the size of a 13-perch plot. The answer was barely one-tenth of an acre. It was upsetting to see the small tract of land designated to support a large family and provide rent to a landlord.

Like many Americans, I heard of the potato famine and knew that waves of immigrants came to the US to escape the ravages of the crop failures from 1845-1852 but I had no idea how it impacted my ancestors. It

---

8 The taxable (or "rateable") value was the income that the property was expected to produce in a year. Annual tax rates for the tenants were often based on the rateable value and could exceed 70% of that value. One pound, five shillings would be worth about $2557 today.

wasn't until I really delved into the history of the famine with Brendan's help that I understood the forces at play in the destruction of Ireland's economy and culture over hundreds of years that allowed the famine to continue its devastation for decades after its height.

In 1841, just prior to the famine, Ireland's census returns show approximately 8.2 million residents in what is now the Republic of Ireland and Northern Ireland combined. The Irish population, through starvation, disease, and emigration, dropped to 6.6 million by the next census in 1851.[9]

What is less well-known is how the English dominated landholdings in Ireland, forcing the Irish to be so dependent on potato crops, and how the Irish Penal Laws severely oppressed the Irish-Catholic population. After Cromwell invaded Ireland in 1649, the English divided Ireland into huge parcels of land and gave them to mostly absentee English landlords, who treated the previous Irish landholders as tenants, from whom rents were due. The English landlord's agents in Ireland subdivided these holdings into tiny parcels of poor-quality land suitable for few crops other than the potato and rented them at exorbitant rates to Irish subsistence farmers like John McGuirk. Failure to make the payments meant eviction with no recourse. The higher quality land, about 75% of English-controlled land, was used to raise a much wider variety of crops, including oats, barley, and wheat, along with livestock, all exported to England even as the Great Famine destroyed the Irish population.[10] At the same time, the draconian 1695 Irish Penal Laws remained in force. Among other things, they restricted education, seized lands, prohibited trade with other countries, banned Catholicism and the Irish language, and demanded a tithe to support Protestant churches.

---

9 "Census 2022: Ireland's population hits record levels," *BBC News*, June 23, 2022, www.bbc.com/news/uk-northern-ireland-61910927, accessed October 30, 2023. The population has still not recovered from the famine. Census 2022 shows that the population has reached 5.1 million people in the Republic of Ireland , and census figures released last month by the NI Statistics and Research Agency (NISRA) show that Northern Ireland's population has grown to just under two million.

10 Jerry Mulvihill, *The Truth about the Irish Famine 1845-1852* (2020), 77-99.

While the famine raged across Ireland from 1845-1852, its effects were felt well into the 1860s when my great-great-grandfather emigrated. "The early 1860s were especially bad years for rural Ireland: unusually wet weather ruined pastures, cash crops, potatoes, and turf, thus injuring graziers [livestock farmers], commercial tillage farmers, subsistence cultivators, and laborers alike. In 1861-64 evictions were 65 percent more numerous than in the preceding four years, and the poor inhabitants of many midland and western counties endured near-famine conditions."[11]

I knew that by the time John Robert McGuirk emigrated in 1861, my great-great-great-grandparents along with their six children had survived the horrors of the famine. They saw neighbors brutally evicted from their homes and left to die of starvation. They did their best to carve out a life on a tiny plot of land where only potatoes grew, besieged by a landlord demanding excessive rent under the threat of eviction with no end in sight. They lived their lives under the severe restrictions of the Irish Penal Laws that ripped away their language and their religion along with their dignity. Once I learned the full story behind the Great Famine, I could understand how a mother, like my great-great-great grandmother Catherine Gervin McGuirk, could endure the loss of her beloved son as he followed the emigration pattern of the famine and sailed to America to start a life free from the pain of living under British rule in Ireland.

Irish emigration did not only occur in the 1800s or involve the United States. Irish emigration continues to this day. Some Irish emigrants have taken a small leap across the Irish Sea where they often settle in Liverpool or further north into Scotland. Canada also proved to be a popular choice with other expatriates heading to Australia or New Zealand to start their lives anew. But wherever the emigrants moved, they took not only their

---

11 Kerby Miller, *Emigrants and Exiles: Ireland and the Irish Exodus to North America* (New York: Oxford University Press, 1985), 360. Evictions estimates range from 250,000 to 500,000.

Irish culture and heritage but also their genetic legacy that forever linked them to their origins in Ireland.

We had one more stop for the day that was related to a tale that Brendan loved to tell me with a promise that when I visited, he would take me to see the exact spot documented in his story. He pointed out that although the folklore, legends, oral history, and place-names offered clues to real giants who once lived in the area, one narrative he came across in his research offered tangible proof. He was keen to show me the place.

To understand why this location stood out to Brendan, we need to go back to the 1830s for a dramatic account of its discovery. In 1824, the English Parliament started a comprehensive survey to map Ireland which resulted in a series of published reports known as the *Ordnance Survey Memoirs of Ireland*. While the stated goal of the project was to survey and map, the project produced much more than maps. Local history and landmarks made their way into the documents, providing an incredible window into the past with details of giant history near the geographic hotspot for the genetic mutation for gigantism.

In the *Ordnance Survey Memoirs of Ireland: Parishes of Co. Londonderry 1, 1830, 1834, 1836*, the surveyor vividly describes an ancient burial ground called Kille Oewn. Located near Magherafelt north of Cookstown, it was known as the oldest Irish burial ground consecrated and registered in Rome. The site was uncovered when a limestone quarry opened near the burial ground in the late 1700s. The surveyor describes what the workers found in the limestone:

> In working the quarry from 1770 to 1815 and overturning the earthy surface that stood above the limestone, they discovered in its bowels an incalculable quantity of every description of human bones, pieces of coffin boards, rings, clasps and nails. Many of the bones were found to be in a tolerable state of preservation and more than ordinary size, particularly thigh, shin

and jaw bones. There was an arm-bone discovered that far exceeded in length and strength any arm-bones ever known to be lifted out of modern graveyards in this country. Also, a skull of so extraordinary a size that it covered down the head and wig of one of the largest men then living in the neighbourhood. Several of the jaw bones were also so large a size that the largest men visiting the quarry could readily replace them outside their fleshy jaws. The thigh, shin bones and teeth were in many instances found as large as those of horses.[12]

Although fascinated by the immense bones, the workers returned the artifacts to the quarry pits, covered them with unwanted stones, and continued extracting the limestone.

When we pulled over to the side of the road and I got out, Brendan pointed to the fenced-in site of the now abandoned quarry, which flooded more than 100 years ago, leveling the ground. There was no sign of the quarry or burial grounds except for chunks of limestone strewn about on the ground. I reached through the fence to pick up a small piece of the white stone flecked with gray. I could see a tiny remnant of a fossilized shell, as I looked down at the ancient rock in my hand. I thought about how the bones of the giant ancestors dug up in the 1830s now rested beneath the earth, hidden in the remains of the quarry near Magherafelt.

---

12 *Ordnance Survey Memoirs of Ireland: Parishes of Co. Londonderry 1, 1830, 1834, 1836,* eds. Angelique Day and Patrick McWilliams, (Institute of Irish, December 31, 1990), 109-110.

CHAPTER 10

# A SENSE OF PLACE

A fter a restful night in a comfy inn just off the town square in Moy, Cherie and I headed out for our last day in County Tyrone. Brendan invited us to spend the day at his home near Dungannon before our drive back to Belfast early the next morning. When we arrived, Brendan's wife Patricia greeted us warmly and led us into their living room where she left us with Brendan who was relaxing in his red recliner watching Gaelic football on the television.

As I looked around the room, I saw vintage family photographs on the wall which reminded me that because they were blood relatives of Brendan on his mother's side, they were relatives of mine even if our connection was in the distant past. I noticed the hefty books on his coffee table that showed his love of Irish history, especially *The Atlas of the Great Irish Famine*. He made a point of showing me the maps in the book, bright color-coded images that detailed the drastic decline in the population of Ireland.

Patricia returned with tea, and we set about chatting about politics, a hot topic in Northern Ireland at the time because County Tyrone native Michelle O'Neill (she attended the same school as Brendan) won the election for the leadership sweeping the Nationalist party Sinn Féin into power for the first time in the 100-year-old history of Northern Ireland.

Brendan sent me upstairs to his library to get a book, telling me to borrow any I liked. His library shelves were packed, with more books in stacks on the floor. Libraries are a window in to someone's mind, and I could see that Brendan's was filled with the Irish language, Celtic myth and legends, genealogy, Ulster history, and the Troubles. I plucked Bernadette Devlin's 1969 autobiography *The Price of My Soul* off the shelf. I was eager to read the Cookstown resident and Irish Republican firebrand's account of the civil rights march from Coalisland to Dungannon, which marked the beginning of the Troubles.

The time flew by, and it seemed like we had just gotten there when Patricia called us to lunch. As I savored her delicious Irish stew, I asked her for her recipe for wheaten bread. I was delighted at how easy it was to relax and enjoy the day. I felt like a long-lost cousin who found her way home.

After lunch, our conversation turned to the next day when Cherie and I planned to drive to Belfast to drop off the rental car and catch a flight to London to meet Professor Korbonits at her laboratory and take a tour of St. Bartholomew's Hospital. Brendan and his son Stephen would be joining us in London making it a homecoming for Brendan who was treated at Barts so many years ago. I was excited about finally meeting her in person and seeing her lab after talking with her via Zoom and spending so much time learning about her research.

All too soon it was time to go. Before we left for the day, Brendan reached out to me with a gift. It was his Gaelic Athletic Association jacket marked with the bright red hand of Ulster on the front. As I tried it on, it felt like a big warm hug. I would remember that feeling when I was at home and was reminded of that cozy day with my newfound family at Brendan's home in County Tyrone.

After our busy trek through Northern Ireland, it was a treat to relax in London on a beautiful day in May seated at a sidewalk table at the Queen's Pub and Dining Room near Regent's Park. Cherie pointed out some makeshift tables festooned in tropical decor along the sidewalk further down the street, a holdover from the pandemic when indoor dining was banned. As we sipped our beers and chatted about our upcoming day at Barts, trendy dog walkers passed by on their way to the park. I told Cherie that Dr. Ben Loughrey and Professor Besser, who was retired, planned to meet with us tomorrow as well. I heard so much about Professor Besser and his distinguished career from Brendan, so I was very curious to meet him.

I already met Dr. Loughrey online when he attended some of our Zoom meetings. An endocrinologist from Belfast with a keen interest in pituitary tumors, he had a temporary fellowship in Professor Korbonits' laboratory at the time. He worked with her previously on a book chapter about hereditary pituitary tumors, including hundreds of germline *AIP* and *GPR101* mutations that potentially lead to symptomatic tumors with geographical links from around the world.[1]

The next morning, Cherie and I took a black cab to the Pret a Manger coffee shop near Charterhouse Square where we would meet up with Brendan, his son Stephen, and Professor Korbonits. While we waited for the others, Cherie asked me what I knew about Professor Korbonits outside her professional expertise. How did a Hungarian endocrinologist wind up at a preeminent hospital in London doing cutting-edge research? I told Cherie that before coming to London I interviewed Professor Korbonits for this book, so I filled her in on what I learned.

Professor Korbonits' story is one of determination, serendipity, and a bit of luck, and it starts in Budapest, Hungary. Both her maternal great grandfather and his eldest son were doctors. She told me that she still has his large 1880 diploma with its big red seal from Franz Joseph Medical University to remind her of her medical roots. Despite her family's history in medicine, at an early age Professor Korbonits had no interest in being a doctor even though her best friend in elementary school wanted to be one. She thought that being a doctor was "very cheesy."

---

1 Paul Benjamin Loughrey and Márta Korbonits, "Genetics of Pituitary Tumors," in *Genetics of Endocrine Diseases and Syndromes*, eds. Peter Igaz and Attila Patócs (Springer International Publishing, 2019), 171-212.

As she got older, biology became a favorite subject. Luckily, advice from her aunt's friend, a biologist, changed her mind when he told her something she remembers to this day. "If you want to be a biologist, be a doctor because as a doctor you can always be a scientist, but if you study biology, you will never be able to be a doctor." She thought that was a very logical argument, and she liked logic. She decided to apply to medical school.

A summer stint working in an asthma ward for children confirmed her decision. She realized, "you would have a child with an asthma attack, and you would inject something, and the asthma would go away and the totally unwell child in a few minutes is smiling and wants to play again. I really enjoyed that." She used that experience to write about the causes of asthma and entered a nationwide biology competition, taking first place and guaranteeing her entry into medical school. "After that, I decided I really liked medicine, and I didn't think it was cheesy anymore."

Endocrinology caught her attention in year two of Semmelweis Medical School. Once again, logic played a role her decision when she noticed that in endocrinology, "something goes up and something goes down, so it is nicely logical." Her 4th year endocrinology Professor Edit Glaz inspired her with her enthusiasm and engaging lectures and convinced her that endocrinology was her path. After graduating with outstanding credentials at the Institute of Pathophysiology, she revamped the undergraduate endocrinology curriculum, which meant learning the latest science and linking it with clinical medicine. When she finished, she knew that she "was totally hooked."

As she developed her medical career in Hungary, the nation was going through tremendous changes as it moved away from its status as a communist Eastern Bloc satellite country. By 1990, the Republic of Hungary had begun; Soviet troops had withdrawn; and Hungary joined other independent nations no longer behind the Iron Curtain. Professor Korbonits left in 1990 when her husband got a job with the BBC World Service in

London. She left behind her home and a country deep in a recession as it worked to establish itself as a democratic nation.

Although she was a junior clinical endocrinologist in Hungary, she could not practice medicine until completing the transfer of her medical credentials to the British system. She obtained a letter of introduction from an endocrinologist in Budapest to give to the dean at St. Bartholomew's Medical School in London. "I mailed that letter, but I never got an answer. I wrote again. Then tried to phone and was advised that Professor Mike Besser, the Head of Endocrinology, had my letter. I phoned his secretary, explained my situation and—this shows how important secretaries can be—she just gave me an appointment and told Professor Besser I needed to be sorted out."

Professor Besser knew that she came from the political turmoil going on in Hungary in the 1990s and that Barts had a tradition of helping doctors from other countries. He also recognized her abilities and admired her determination. Normally, doctors from abroad were financially independent with resources to fund their labs, but he decided to give her a chance to help with research already in progress in the endocrinology department and found the money to pay her salary and other expenses.

He was right to have faith in her. By the early 2000s, Professor Korbonits established herself at Barts as a clinical academic researcher in endocrinology with a prestigious Medical Research Council Clinician Scientist fellowship, which eventually led to her research in genetic gigantism that was the subject of the 2011 research paper that I found online.

I knew that by 2020 she published more than 200 original papers, but I told my sister for me the most important thing she did was to continue being a practicing physician not solely an academic researcher. She chose to connect her academic research to her work as a practicing physician by searching for meaningful solutions to help her patients to cope with some of medicine's rarest diseases.

As I finished my story, I looked up to see Brendan and Stephen and waved them over to join us. When Stephen went up to order coffee for them, I saw Professor Korbonits breeze in the door. I flashbacked to when I first learned about her London-based research, and I imagined that she was a stodgy British researcher unlikely to welcome my inquiries. I learned just how wrong my stereotype of a British researcher could be when I met her online and saw her lively and inviting face framed by a neat chestnut bob. Meeting her in person only confirmed what I discovered during our online meetings. She radiated enthusiasm, and she was eager to show us her lab. We hurriedly finished our coffee and set off for her laboratory about 10 minutes away.

As we walked along the streets of London in the 21st century, we moved through a modern cityscape of fast-moving double-decker buses, blinking city lights, and fashionable restaurants, but what fascinated me was that we were surrounded by landmarks where 18th century Charles Byrne and Dr. John Hunter once walked.

I knew we were near the Victorian-era Smithfield Market, a poultry and meat market that stretches for four city blocks and is still in active commerce today. The main Central Market building is an enormous red brick, two-story structure with iron columns and wrought iron walls painted magenta and teal with a delicate glass and iron filigree domed roof. The building is a far cry from the open-air meat market that once existed on the site during Charles Byrne's time with its cacophony of thousands of sheep and cattle kept in fenced pens.

As we neared the hospital, I could see a street sign for Cloth Fair, an area once home to the raucous Bartholomew Fair where Charles Byrne displayed himself as one of the Fair's many curiosities. As Byrne made his way around the Fair, he could have looked up at the statue of King Henry VIII found atop the gateway at the entrance to the hospital grounds. Erected in 1702, the commemorative entryway marks one of the most important events in the hospital's history. Instead of closing the monastery and St. Bartholomew's Hospital in 1637 during the Dissolution of the

Monasteries,[2] King Henry VIII bowed to public pressure and granted the monastery and its hospital to the city of London under Royal Charter, preventing its closure.

St. Bartholomew's Hospital itself would have been a familiar sight in the 1700s. By 1769, the hospital consisted of four buildings that formed a square around a central courtyard, a design in place during Dr. John Hunter's time. The central courtyard is a quiet refuge amid the commotion of modern London, and I recognized its ornate 1859 central fountain as the place where Brendan and Professor Korbonits first met in the Charles Byrne documentary.

Even the land itself where the original hospital was built stands out for its unusual history. Charterhouse Square is the location of what is believed to be the largest mass grave in London during the Black Death (1347-1351) with an estimated 50,000 bodies interred at the burial ground and its plague pit.[3] It may have once been a burial ground, but today it is an academic hub comprised of the campus of Queen Mary University of London and research organizations such as the William Harvey Research Institute, which houses the Centre for Endocrinology where Professor Korbonits works.

We entered the door to the Centre, and we wound our way through the maze-like hallways on the way to the conference room where we planned to meet up with Dr. Loughrey and Professor Besser. We passed by a warren of rooms filled with lab benches, centrifuges, blue gloves, and purple-capped specimen vials. We paused at one of the doors and peered in at the white lab-coat-clad researcher who glanced up at us from her bench and smiled. Professor Korbonits told me that she was the person

---

2 The Dissolution of the Monasteries (1536-1541) occurred when Henry VIII closed Catholic monasteries, priories, convents, and friaries in England, Wales, and Ireland, seizing their assets to establish the Church of England during the English Reformation.

3 Ben Johnson, "The Reputed Plague Pits of London," *Historic UK*, https://www.historic-uk.com/HistoryMagazine/DestinationsUK/LondonPlaguePits/.

who analyzed my son's tumor specimen. It was great to be able to thank her directly for her work.

We continued and met a few of the other scientists who bustled around us, intent on their work. They looked up in curiosity when Professor Korbonits paused to tell us a bit about their research. I thanked them for their work and identified myself a few times by the code number assigned to me to maintain my anonymity in their database which drew a delighted chuckle. I am sure that they spend countless hours during their research staring at data classified by code numbers, so it was refreshing to see one of their patients standing before them instead of just a number on a page.

One room stood out in my mind. It was a small, darkened room packed with electronic devices, cables, and computer equipment. A large computer monitor displayed a colorful image of a cell's structure, illuminating the room in a blue and red glow. The researcher's gaze was fixed on the screen as he peered into the underlying cell structure displayed in front of him. I realized that the researchers in Professor Korbonits' lab worked on many different levels from microscopic cell anatomy to the macrocosm of data sets with extensive family trees going back generations.

Before we went into the conference room, I noticed a large display of photographs, 68 headshots portraying each of the scientists involved in the Centre for Endocrinology and its research. I paused to take in each of their faces, and I hoped that they realized how important their work was to the patients they might never see but whose lives have been changed for the better by their work.

As we sat down in the conference room to wait, Dr. Loughrey joined us. Professor Korbonits asked if we had any questions. I didn't have time to respond because I looked up to see a distinguished older gentleman enter the room. Professor Besser had arrived. I didn't know what to expect. I heard that he was very direct and spoke his mind, so I didn't know what he would make of me and my sister, the Americans sitting before him. I knew that he was a recognized professor and physician, widely admired for his clinical expertise and ground-breaking contributions to endocrinology. I also knew that he was an extremely skilled and accomplished leader when as the Chief Executive of Barts in the early 1990s, he stared down the conservative forces trying to shutter Barts, preventing its closure.

I could tell by his demeanor that he was no stranger to this academic environment as he set aside his walking cane and eased into his chair. We exchanged pleasantries and then he said something to me that I didn't expect. "Welcome to the Barts family." I was momentarily stunned by what he said, touched that he went out of his way to make me feel comfortable. Then I realized that I had indeed stepped into a "family" by being a part of the research going on at Barts. I belonged here, and I felt supported by the research going on in Professor Korbonits' lab. I knew that I was one tiny data point in an enormous database, but I felt a real sense of security knowing that so many researchers were taking seriously the difficulties of having a rare disease like gigantism.

With our group assembled, we headed out the door for lunch at the Smith Restaurant across from the Smithfield Market. The food was exceptional. I made a point of sitting next to Professor Besser so that I could get to know him better and found myself hanging on to his every word. He was very congenial and chatty, talking about his life as an emeritus professor and how he played a killer game of croquet with his fellow retirees. I asked him what brought him to St. Bartholomew's Hospital in the first place.

Professor Besser told me that he was the grandson of Jewish refugees who escaped the pogroms in Poland and settled in the East End of London. He grew up south of London in Morden during World War II until his family evacuated further south to Hove after bombs fell on the recreation ground at his school. No one in his family had ever gone to a university, yet he excelled in school, his hard work and dedication winning him a spot in St. Bartholomew's Medical School in 1954. He spent his entire career at Barts.

He told me that he was grateful for what Barts had given him, but it was clear that he had given back through his dedication and service. His scientific accomplishments at Barts were world-renowned, but that was only part of his contribution. He used his research to benefit his patients when he directly linked his discoveries to patient care in his clinic. This is probably his greatest legacy, his belief that the true worth of scientific research lies in its clinical application.

I could see how his legacy lives through the leading endocrinologists he trained, like Professor Korbonits, who continue to practice at Barts today. I asked him what he saw in Professor Korbonits that led him to offer her a job so long ago. He replied that although she was a junior clinician, she was eager to learn, and he recognized her abilities. Perhaps, he also saw in her the same thing that I saw when I first met her online—the light of enthusiasm, determination, and curiosity in her eyes.

After lunch, we headed over to the historic part of St. Bartholomew's Hospital. As we were walking, I thought about what I learned when I read up on its early history before coming to London. I was fascinated by the story that began 900 years ago when a favorite court jester of Henry I named Rahere decided to go on a pilgrimage to Rome. While there, he contracted malaria. The monks from a small hospital attached to a church dedicated to St. Bartholomew nursed him as he got sicker and sicker. According to legend, Rahere was close to death, feverish and in pain, when the winged Beast of the Apocalypse appeared to him. As he looked up at the vision, he begged God to allow him to live so that he could return to England to build a hospital also dedicated to St. Bartholomew that would provide the same compassionate care he was receiving. The creature disappeared, and Rahere's fever broke. Rahere was saved.

As soon as he recovered, Rahere hurried back to England. During the trip, he was again overcome with a vision. This time it was St. Bartholomew who told him to build the church in Smithfield. When Rahere told Henry I of his divine visions, the king gave him land in Smithfield to build the

Priory Church of St. Bartholomew the Great, which eventually became the site of St. Bartholomew's Hospital.

When we reached the hospital grounds, Will Palin, Chief Executive Officer for Barts Heritage Trust was on hand to take us on the tour of the hospital's North Wing, which was completed in 1734. As part of the celebration of the 900th anniversary of the founding of St. Bartholomew's Hospital, the Barts Heritage Trust agreed to repair the North Wing's Great Hall with Palin leading the conservation and fundraising efforts. The £22 million project is slated for completion in 2025. I was excited to take the tour because I read about the building's architectural beauty, but also because I thought it would give me insight into the culture of the hospital from its earliest days in 1123 to the present. Brendan told me many times that the philosophy of health at Barts was pivotal to its success in treating patients.

As Mr. Palin opened the door and welcomed us into the first floor of the North Wing, we were greeted by a massive Georgian era staircase with intricately carved wooden banisters and delicate scrollwork, leading up to the Great Hall. We ascended to the top to view the two magnificent paintings that framed the staircase and extended to the ceiling. Painted by William Hogarth in the 1730s, the works illustrate the biblical tale of the Good Samaritan who rescued a man after a violent attack and the story of how Christ healed a lame man at the Pool of Bethesda.

I gazed at the paintings with their larger-than-life figures and noted how the paintings reflect the hospital's healing culture and spiritual origins. The Good Samaritan tenderly applies a healing oil to the chest wounds of the fallen man while the man's bandaged arm rests comfortably on a rock. The Good Samaritan has created a restorative place of calm with his horse nearby ready to take the man to an inn where he can get further help.

In the Pool of Bethesda, Jesus and the lame man take the central focus of the painting, but the other figures in the work are what draws my eye. One elderly man leans on a crutch, his belly bloated and his cheeks sunken. Another man, his head wrapped with a cloth stares out with yellowed eyes while a woman clutches her breast in pain with her emaciated arm. The people depicted are not society's elite. They are everyday ordinary people with conditions such as tuberculosis, jaundice, and breast cancer. The images are so vivid that the paintings are still in use as an educational tool with medical students. Using patients from the hospital as models, Hogarth captured the pain and suffering, yet hope of those coming to St. Bartholomew's for treatment.

We turned from the painting and walked through a short dark hallway behind us and into the Great Hall. Like magic, the room opened before us with its bright vaulted ceilings covered in ornate plaster medallions and gold leaf embellishments, elaborate crown moldings, and marble fireplaces. On the walls, giant wooden plaques dating back to 1547 with the names of 3,000 benefactors inscribed in gold letters surrounded us. Henry

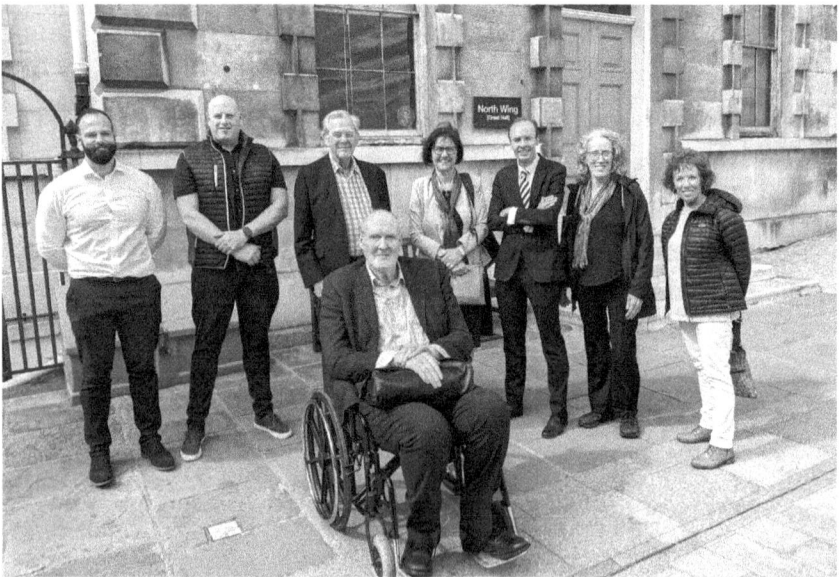

From the left, Dr. Loughrey, Stephen Holland, Professor Besser, Brendan, Professor Korbonits, Will Palin, Colleen, and Cherie

VIII peered down on us from his stained-glass window, bringing multi-hued light into the space. I could feel the weight of 900 years of history and was amazed at how St. Bartholomew's survived from the Middle Ages, through the 1666 Great Fire of London and the Blitz of World War II, and into the 21st century.

After visiting the hall, we descended the staircase and gathered outside for a group photo. I looked back at the North Wing, and I felt fortunate to find this place with its historic legacy of healing. I was also grateful for the people who stood with me—Brendan, Cherie, Professor Besser, Professor Korbonits, and Dr. Loughrey—and helped me through my genetic journey. I was flying home the next day, and it was hard to say goodbye to them. I knew I would see my sister again soon after our trip, but I wasn't sure if I would ever see Professor Besser again. I hoped that I could keep in touch with Professor Korbonits and Dr. Loughrey. For Brendan, I knew that the connection between us was deep and that he was only a video chat or phone call away.

# CHAPTER 11

# THE TRAVELING GENE

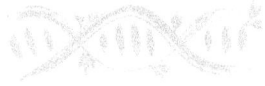

O ver the next year, I often reflected on how much I learned about genetics and its impact on me. Before I knew about Professor Korbonits' work, the only thing I knew about genetics was what I learned in my high school science class in the 1970s. Genetics seemed placid, orderly, and predictable like a quiet pond. It was only after I began to look at my genetic heritage that I understood how forceful the flow could be. In some families, the genetic mutation rippled through a large family tree, unnoticed, kept in the stream of life by genetic carriers. In other families, the genetic mutation roared through their family tree like a flooded river, powerful and dynamic, causing multiple family members to develop a pituitary tumor and become symptomatic. For me, the genetic mutation got caught up in the ocean currents that brought ships from Ireland across the sea to America in the 1800s and survived for four generations before finding me.

After I returned home from my travels, I continued to search for stories about people with the *AIP* genetic mutation in the hope of finding other families affected by gigantism. I was particularly interested in how the genetic mutation moved out into the world following immigration patterns. I asked Professor Korbonits if she knew anyone else with the *AIP* mutation whose family history showed how the gene traveled out from the geographic hotspot into the world like mine did. She told me that she had a patient in Scotland, and she would ask him if he was willing to talk with me about his experience. After getting his permission, she gave me his email address. I was delighted when he answered that he was happy to chat.

When Phil Burnside first appeared on my computer screen during our video meeting in April 2023, I was struck by his open, welcoming demeanor and his warm sienna skin that revealed his West Indies heritage. He didn't look like a stereotypical Scotsman; however, his melodious Scottish accent immediately placed him firmly in my mind as the Scotsman he is. I quickly realized that he was as eager to talk with me as I was with him, as he set about telling me his story. In the telling, I learned just how far the *AIP* gene mutation can travel beyond its geographic origins.

Phil was born in Edinburgh, Scotland in 1970. "My father was from the West Indies, and my mother was from a place called Paisley near Glasgow. I was adopted out at the age of nine months, and then I moved to Coatbridge [in Scotland] where I've been basically my whole life." Phil told me how grateful he was to have a wonderful adoptive family and "a phenomenal upbringing in comparison to what it could have been." Even with the best of luck, his life still proved to be difficult as a Black child growing up in Scotland with a White family in the 1970s. "There weren't many Black people around in the UK, especially in Scotland. That was a challenge right there in itself. I think that was part of the reason my mother made the decision to adopt me out. She was quite young. I was very blessed with the family that looked after me."

Although his adoptive family was very open with him about his adoption, he did not have any medical information or details about his biological parents. At times, he was curious about his biological parents, but he didn't feel a need to find them given his happy home life. "Being adopted, you go through life forever wondering. There are always some question marks on you. Where did you come from? Who are you? They're all natural questions to ask. Any time your family history comes up, on doctor forms or whatever, you have to say I don't know. Through my life I was very much thinking about it and on a few occasions, I thought, I'm going to do it, I'm going to look and find my natural mother, but I just put it off."

He told me that his son was born in 1997, and that his son developed a pituitary tumor when he was probably around age 10. However, he wasn't diagnosed with the tumor until he was 15 years old. "At this point, his mother and I were not together anymore, and I was still in Glasgow, but he was living with his mother in Brighton south of London, so he was under England's National Health Service. It took a long time to get it diagnosed. It really was an odyssey."

Phil attributes the difficulty in getting a diagnosis for his son to several factors. "Doctors were just saying that he suffered from headaches or growing pains or some sort of thing." Phil also thought that it was because both of his son's parents were quite tall. "His mother is about six feet tall (183 cm), and I'm quite tall myself, about five eleven (180 cm), so the doctors also thought with tall parents, he'd be tall. Two tall parents you would expect him to be at least six feet two or three (~190 cm)." It wasn't until his son started growing rapidly—shooting up more than six inches (15 cm) in less than six months—that the doctors focused on why his son was going through an accelerated growth spurt rather than just attributing the growth to puberty. "It's just potluck [which doctors] you get and how engaged they are in terms of understanding the pathways that people have to go on [to get a diagnosis] and what is the direct pathway." Getting a diagnosis often depends on getting the right doctor at the right time.

Phil also credits his son's mother for her persistence in getting answers to what was going on with their son. As his son's symptoms worsened, she worked hard to find the right specialists. Her determination led to the correct diagnosis. "By then he was just growing and growing and growing. He outgrew his beds. He had some sight loss. And there was the association of all the other pains and eye problems and all these other things that were coming along. His mum had to push and pursue it to get things sorted out. In the end, it worked out to be a good thing that she pushed because my son ended up in the endocrinology department with a well-regarded endocrinologist at King's College Hospital. Only when he was over six foot seven (201 cm) did he get the diagnosis." With a proper diagnosis, doctors developed a successful treatment plan of surgery and radiotherapy to eliminate his pituitary tumor and a plan for his continued care. At six feet eleven inches tall (211 cm), he finally stopped growing.

Given that his son's tumor started when he was young, the doctors recommended that his son undergo genetic testing for the *AIP* gene mutation in the hope of finding the cause of the pituitary tumor. When the testing came back positive, Phil assumed it was his son's mother who was the carrier. "I thought it had to be his mother, but she just laughed at me and said, 'you're the one, you're the one who carries the gene.' I thought, what? How would that be possible?" Guessing which parent is the carrier can be a point of contention, but the solution is straightforward: take the test.

First, Phil needed to convince his Scottish doctor to write the order for the test. Because the *AIP* mutation is rare, it can be a challenge to get the testing done because a general practitioner is unlikely to know about the mutation and its impact. My sister had a similar challenge when she went to her doctor to get the order for testing and needed to provide the information on the mutation so that the doctor felt comfortable ordering the needed DNA test. "I had to go to the GP and say, you need to send me for the test. It wasn't even something I could fully understand and explain, and the GP had never heard of this gene before. I was fortunate that I had a GP that listened and ordered the test."

Phil was referred to a genetics clinic in Glasgow for the test. After a few weeks, Phil had his answer. "They told me that I had it. I was the carrier."

His thoughts turned to his daughter. "And that started the question of what about my daughter, who was about eight years old. The idea was just to get her checked out from an early point, and if there was something there, we could do something quickly about it." His daughter was tested, and it turned out that she had the defective gene. "So, she is now under the care of the doctors in Glasgow, who are watching her closely. She's in her teens now. We can see my daughter growing, and we just can't wait for her to stop. Whether or not the acromegaly comes later we'll see. But so far so good; she's healthy."

Phil had long wondered about his biological parents but didn't feel an intense desire to connect with them. Finding out that he had the genetic mutation changed his mind. He wanted to learn his medical history. It was obvious that his adoptive parents were not the carriers. Phil was very skeptical that it was his father because he was from the West Indies with no known connection to Ireland. Although he didn't know his mother, he knew that she was Scottish because he was adopted in Scotland. Being Scottish also made it more likely that she had Irish ancestors. He suspected that she was the carrier who passed the gene on to him, but without the testing, it wasn't possible to answer the question of who carried the gene. "We had no idea where the gene came from, so I reached out to the adoption society that looked after me."

Phil had to wait for the life-changing answer to his question: who is my mother? After several weeks, the adoption agency contacted him. They found his mother. She was living in Australia, and she was willing to connect with him.

Their connection began with a few phone calls during which Phil learned that his mother moved from Scotland to Australia shortly after giving him up for adoption, where she started a family and had five children. Only a few months later, they were able to meet in Glasgow. "She was already planning to be there in three months, so we met up then. I had the very surreal moment of meeting someone for the first time, who was actually my mother. My siblings had no idea that I even existed."

His world shifted to one that now included his mother and five half-siblings. But he still needed to answer the second question: who is my father? He didn't have to wait long for an answer. "So, a few months later, I found my father, and he had ten children. I went from being the youngest in my adoptive family [of three children] to being the oldest one in my natural mother and father's families. So, it ended up that I was one of eighteen children. That number is just bonkers."

His mother was curious about why he decided to reach out to her after so many years. "When I told my natural mother about the gene, she was stunned by the whole thing." He explained to her about the importance of knowing who had the gene in their extended family, finding anyone with medical problems related to a pituitary tumor caused by the gene, and monitoring their family tree for anyone who might be at risk in the future. "I told her that I decided to find her because if there was anyone else out there that could potentially have this gene and could avoid having their life impacted by it, then I wanted to do that."

Both parents were tested, which revealed that she was the carrier. The next step was to draw up his mother's family tree or pedigree, determine who was at risk, and begin cascade genetic testing of the family members who might carry the gene. Creating the family tree also revealed an important geographical connection. "The interesting part was when we were looking at [my mother's family pedigree], we realized that her mother, my grandmother, came from quite close to the geographic area in Northern Ireland where the gene originated. So that was quite a link there."

Given the difficulty that I encountered when I tried to get my blood relatives at risk for the gene tested, I was quite interested in how successful Phil was in getting his long-lost relatives to agree to be tested, especially given that none of them appeared to have acromegaly or gigantism. The first round of testing included his mother's five children, her three brothers, and her one sister. All five of his half-siblings were tested, and three out of five were found to have the *AIP* genetic mutation. When the children of the three half-siblings who tested positive were in turn tested, none carried the gene.

His mother's sister opted out of testing because she had no symptoms and no children to pass on the gene, while two out of three of his mother's brothers were tested. One of them tested positive. His children were then tested, and his daughter proved to have the defective gene. She also found out that she had a pituitary tumor. "She's quite tall, but she has no other effects whatsoever. She was so delighted to have the information to know what was going on." Phil told me how his experience with getting his family tested proved how important it is to get accurate medical information out there. "I think information is key. There's a certain degree of people who say what will be, will be, and you can't do anything about it. And that is probably once it's too late. It is getting ahead of the game for people who've got medical issues, isn't it?" Phil succeeded in giving his newly discovered biological family the information they needed to understand the potential impact of having the gene mutation, and they responded by getting the testing that they needed.

As Phil and I came to the end of our video chat, we both reflected on just how much our definition of family expanded through the experience of having a genetic mutation and tracing that mutation through our family trees. Phil now knew his biological family and found his place in that family tree. I felt I added Phil as another cousin to mine. We have a biological connection even though it may have been hundreds if not thousands of years in the past. Knowing that we both shared the same *AIP* genetic mutation meant that we are kin. We also have the shared experience of our families being affected by the *AIP* gene mutation linked to the same area in Northern Ireland between the Sperrin Mountains and Lough Neagh. The geographic hotspot was like the headwaters of a river that caused the gene to flow out into the world, meandering its way to America, Scotland, and Australia. Our families may have moved from Ireland, but because we carry the genetic mutation, we can always look to those headwaters and call Northern Ireland our home.

# CHAPTER 12

# GIGANTISM
# AROUND THE WORLD

A s the pandemic waned throughout 2023, I continued to meet with Brendan, and I relished the times that I delved into the folklore and legends surrounding giants in the north. I felt that my personal questions about the *AIP* mutation were answered, and I had a firm understanding of the Northern Ireland variant that can cause genetic gigantism. Nevertheless, I knew that I still had a lot to learn, when Professor Korbonits pointed out to me that Northern Ireland is not the only country affected by genetic gigantism, and the Arg304stop mutation is not the only mutation that leads to gigantism.

Just as I explored the land of giants in Northern Ireland online, I set off on another virtual expedition in search of giants—this time to discover others with genetic gigantism found throughout the world.

I needed to prepare myself for that virtual journey by learning about how researchers point to the location of a particular gene on the human genome when discussing a genetic mutation. The human genome has 23 pairs of chromosomes, each containing a varied number of genes, so first, the scientist refers to the gene's location in the genome based on the chromosome where it resides. The *AIP* gene is located on chromosome 11.

Next, the researcher states a number to show where the mutation lies along that gene and adds the base pair changes as letters. In the case of the

Northern Ireland mutation, the genetic mutation is located at c.910C>T, meaning at the 910th base pair, which changed from a cytosine to a thymine.[1] The researcher then puts in the amino acid number where the change is located and notes how it changed. In the case of the Northern Ireland mutation, the 304th amino acid, normally an arginine, is changed to a stop codon so it is referred to as an Arg304Stop mutation.

I also needed to understand that certain places in the DNA change more easily than others. One such place is the CpG site, where a cytosine is followed by a guanine on one side of the DNA ladder. The *AIP* gene has several such sites. For reasons not fully understood, one of these sites at the 304 location is easily broken (spontaneously mutated) on the gene. This means that there is a higher rate of spontaneous mutation at the 304 location than at other locations along the *AIP* gene. This can happen independently to different people in different countries. It also means that one person with an Arg304Stop gene mutation is not necessarily related to another person with a 304 mutation because they could each have had a different ancestor who was the first to have a Arg304Stop mutation.

So, I now had some understanding of how scientists talk with precision about a gene mutation and narrow it down to a very specific location on the genome. But how do researchers know the difference between one Arg304Stop mutation and another? The answer is microsatellite markers.

Microsatellites are short, repeated sequences of DNA found along a chromosome. These repeated sequences are passed down and are distinct in each genetic line, creating a signature pattern of microsatellites near a 304 gene mutation. Researchers use those signature patterns to figure out whether someone shares a common ancestor who initially had the 304

1 The exact scientific finding was that the Irish variant was a missense mutation due to a base pair change at the 910th base pair of the *AIP* gene, cytosine to thymine (C>T) resulting in a change of the code (triplet base pair CGA) for one of the amino acids, the 304th amino acid of *AIP* protein arginine, to a stop code (TGA). A stop codon causes the protein that is created by the *AIP* gene to be shorter than it should be. Scientists use a coding system to indicate exactly where a mutation occurs in a gene. In this case, it is called at the gene level 910C>T and at the protein level Arg304Stop mutation of the *AIP* gene.

genetic mutation. These wonderous tiny bits of DNA are what link me, Brendan, Niamh, Laura, Phil, and Charles Byrne together as a clan, reaching back in time to one single person who had a spontaneous 304 mutation that was passed down the blood line to us.

My fascination with giants only grew as I learned that the *AIP* mutation at the 304 spot is not solely linked to the geographic location in Northern Ireland. There are others with a 304 mutation different than mine. What was even more intriguing to me was that many of these countries that have proven to be geographic hotspots, like Northern Ireland, have their own rich folklore, legends, and mythology about giants similar to the tales of the Irish giant Fionn Mac Cumhaill. There are also stories about giants from the past who once lived in the area, with historic descriptions that indicate their gigantism might be related to known genetic mutations found in that area.

Mexico, for example, has a cohort of modern-day giants that have been tested and found to have a Arg304Stop mutation distinct from the Northern Ireland version.[2] When I researched Mexico's giant mythology, I needed to go back in time to when the Conquistadors explored and conquered Mexico. As they went from the Baja Peninsula south, they heard Aztec legends of the Quinametzin, or the Giant People, and how they built the colossal ruins found in Mexico. Their gargantuan leader Xelhua is said to have climbed the mountain of Tlaloc to survive a primordial flood that wiped out all but the Quinametzin. In gratitude for being saved, he built the Great Pyramid at Cholula, the largest pyramid in the world, a structure that dates back more than 2,000 years. There is also the tale of the warrior Tzilcatzin, who stood over ten feet (304 cm) tall and fought back against the invading Spaniards by throwing stones to repel the invaders.

In the 16th century, the Spanish missionary José de Acosta settled in Mexico City in 1586 where he collected tales of the civilization and

---

2 Claudia Ramírez-Rentería et al., "*AIP* mutations in young patients with acromegaly and the Tampico Giant: the Mexican experience," *Endocrine* 53, no. 3 (2016): 402-411.

religion of the Aztecs which he documented in his work *The Natural & Moral History of the Indies.* "When I was in Mexico, in the year of our Lord one thousand five hundred eighty six, they found one of those giants buried in one of our farms, which we call Jesus del Monte, of whom they brought a tooth to be seen, which (without augmenting) was as big as the fist of a man, and, according to this, all the rest was proportionate, which I saw and admired at his deformed greatness."[3] I wonder if these Mexican giants of legend and history in the country are related to the giants that live in Mexico today. Further research may one day find a link.

Italy is another country that has been found to have its own Arg304Stop mutation that causes gigantism and a rich history of giant lore. For example, the city Messina in northeast Sicily celebrates its giant mythological founders—the lovers Mata and Grifone. The legend of Mata and Grifone dates back almost 1000 years and weaves a tale of the gigantic pirate named Grifone who falls in love with a beautiful Messinian girl on one of his raids. She rebuffs him because she is disturbed that he is a pirate. When he gives up his life as a buccaneer to win her over, she begins a passionate love affair with him. Tradition holds that their children are the founders of Messina. Today, revelers dance the *Ballo dei Giganti* to a tarantella rhythm as they move through the streets, following colossal papier mâché and wooden statues of their beloved founders.

What really caught my attention as I investigated the roots of gigantism in Italy was an article in the journal *Medical Hypotheses,* which focuses on possible medical diagnoses based on historical records instead of direct examination of a patient. The authors investigated accounts of Maximus Thrax (ca. AD 173-238) who was thought to be one of the tallest men in history for information about his medical and physical condition. Classical sources describe Maximinus as a massive man with enormous

---

3 Joseph de Acosta, *History of the Indies, Vol. II*, translated by Edward Grimston (New York: Burt Franklin, 1970), 453-454.

hands, prominent jaw and forehead, coarse facial features, and a large nose who drank and ate huge quantities and sweated profusely—all symptoms of someone with a pituitary tumor and gigantism. The researchers then analyzed accounts of his son Gaius Iulius Versus Maximus who appeared to be affected by the same disorder, given how contemporary sources described him similarly to his father. The article has pictures of the coins minted at the time of their reign, which show their faces in profile. I could see my face in theirs because my profile is so similar, with the prominent nose and chin of someone with acromegaly or gigantism. Their article concluded that both men most likely had gigantism.

> Although no genetic analysis can be performed on long-lost mortal remains, the available historical sources and the iconographic representations allow us to reasonably postulate that Maximinus Thrax may well have had a mutation in the *AIP* gene, which was inherited by his son Gaius Iulius Verus Maximus.[4]

While the *AIP* gene is easily mutated at the 304 location, the 304 location is not the only area on the *AIP* gene that can be mutated. There are over 100 different mutations that have been detected on the *AIP* gene that can cause gigantism. As I mentioned previously, in 2006 Finnish scientists identified an *AIP* mutation that can cause genetic gigantism at the Gln14 position on the *AIP* gene.[5] The gene runs in Finnish families with roots in the Kainuu region, an area known for its giant heritage and folklore.

Like the Northern Ireland's tourism slogan "Embrace the Giant Spirit" that I encountered when I visited Belfast, the Kainuu region in

---

4  Emanuele Armocida, et al., "Hereditary acromegalic gigantism in the family of Roman Emperor Maximinus Thrax," *Medical Hypotheses* 136 (2020): 109525.

5  Outi Vierimaa et al., "Pituitary adenoma predisposition caused by germline mutations in the *AIP* gene," *Science* 312, no. 5777 (May 26, 2006): 1228-1230.

Finland has a similar tourism advertisement, billing itself as the "Land of Giants." The area boasts giant legends and exceptionally tall men who were born or once lived in the area, particularly in the municipality of Paltamo. Finland's mythology is rich with tales of giant creatures such as the Kalevanpoika, who like Fionn Mac Cumhaill of Irish fame, shape the land by cutting down forests and destroying meadows. Another is the giant Antero Vipunen who sleeps underground. Once awakened, he casts powerful spells and devours those who stir him from his slumber.

The Kainuu region is home to one of the world's tallest men to have ever lived. Finland's Väinö Myllyrinne was born in 1909 in Helsinki, but his mother was from Paltamo in the Kainuu region. He entered the Finnish Defence Forces in 1929 when he was 20 years old, standing 7 feet, 3 inches (218 cm) tall. After leaving the military, he travelled around Europe as a professional wrestler and circus performer. When he was 30 years old, he served in the Finnish Army during the Winter War of 1939 when the Soviet Union invaded Finland. After the war, Myllyrinne began to grow again, and by time he was 40 years old he measured 8 feet, 3 inches (251 cm) tall. He died in 1963 when he was 54 years old, an advanced age for someone with gigantism.

What was most interesting to me about Myllyrinne is that there is a very short film of him shot in 1935 available online, documenting what it was like for someone so tall to simply walk down a street and get on a boat. Those around him barely come to his shoulder, and as he reaches out to shake hands with a policeman, it is clear just how massive his hands and feet are in comparison. When he strides down the gangplank onto the boat, he bends over at the waist and stoops low to enter the housing on the deck. The film finishes with him standing on the stern of the boat, waving to those on shore, surrounded by what appear to be miniature people.[6]

My research took me to Mexico, Italy, and Finland, but it was time

---

6 "Väinö Myllyrinne le géant finnois," (July 29, 1935), https://www.youtube.com/watch?v=U_qjXt9T3kQ.

to look closer to home in the United States when I came across the person widely regarded as the tallest man ever to have lived: Robert Wadlow of Alton, Illinois.

The *AIP* gene, located on chromosome 11, is well known as a cause of gigantism when mutated, but the 11th chromosome is not the only location for genetic mutations that lead to gigantism. The *GPR101* gene is found on the X chromosome and when it is mutated, it can lead to a pituitary tumor that results in X-linked acro-gigantism (X-LAG). X-LAG is an extremely rare and severe form of gigantism that begins in infancy. Those affected are usually born with normal weight and height, but very quickly after birth, they experience rapid and excessive growth.

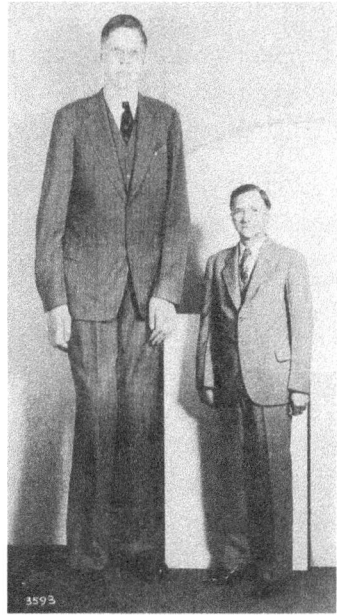

Robert Wadlow and his father, 1937

Although genetic testing was not available when Wadlow was born in 1918, doctors believe that Wadlow had X-LAG, based on his published medical history, symptoms, and physical characteristics.

> Parsing these historical reports and some accompanying scientific observations reveals information indicating that many of the tallest patients in history had an early childhood-onset gigantism phenotype that is highly reminiscent of X-LAG syndrome. As shown in Table 3, these cases [including Wadlow] occurred against a background of a normal family history and, in some, a pituitary pathology was demonstrable.[7]

---

7 Albert Beckers et al., "X-linked acrogigantism syndrome: clinical profile and therapeutic responses," *Endocrine-Related Cancer* 22, no. 3 (2015): 353-367, see Table 3, https://erc.bioscientifica.com/view/journals/erc/22/3/353.xm.

It is easy to see why scientists think that Wadlow had X-LAG syndrome. He was an average newborn, measuring 20 inches (51 cm) and weighing 8 pounds, 5 ounces (3.8 kg), but by the time he was one year old, he was 3 feet 6 inches (107 cm) tall and weighed 45 pounds (20.4 kg). He continued to grow, and four years later, he was as tall as an average man at 5 feet 6.5 inches (169 cm) and weighed 140 pounds (65.5 kg). His growth hormone continued unchecked, and he grew unabated through his adolescence and young adulthood. By his death in 1940, he measured 8 feet 11.1 inches (272 cm) tall and weighed 439 pounds (199 kg). He was only 22 years old.

For his entire life, it was a struggle to move through the world. As a child, he couldn't fit into a regular school desk, and his clothes needed to be custom made. Shoes were particularly difficult to find until the International Shoe Company began to provide free shoes in exchange for Wadlow going on a promotional tour for the company. He traveled to more than 800 towns and 41 states in a car his father adapted so that he could sit in the back seat with his legs stretched out to where the front seat once was. He needed two hotel beds placed end to end to be able to sleep, and ceiling light fixtures were a constant threat. It was even a challenge to sit down, given that few chairs were available to accommodate his weight.[8]

I came across a documentary filmed in 1975 that offers a fascinating look into Wadlow's life through film footage and interviews with classmates, teachers, neighbors, and colleagues who knew him. His teacher mentioned how tiny the paper and pencil looked in his huge hands as a child and how it was nearly impossible for him to write. His manager pointed out how challenging life on the road was for Wadlow while he was on promotional tour for the shoe company. Sometimes a customer came up and kicked him in the leg from behind, thinking it was all a joke and

---

8 Frederick Drimmer, *Born Different: Amazing Stories of Very Special People* (New York: Bantam Skylark Book, 1991), 49-50.

that Wadlow really was on stilts. It is sad to watch the film footage and see how difficult it was for Wadlow to move. Nonetheless, it is heartening to see his constant smile and his sunny personality, characteristics often mentioned in the film interviews.[9]

In 1936, he set off on a tour with Ringling Brothers Circus when he was 18 years old. Despite his limited mobility, he never used a wheelchair; instead, he relied on leg braces and canes to help him move around. He had little sensation in his feet and legs, so he did not feel the blisters forming on his feet until one became infected. Unable to be accommodated at the hospital due to his enormous size, he stayed near the hospital at a hotel where beds could be pushed together to make him more comfortable. The doctors tried blood infusions and emergency surgery, to no avail. Wadlow died from complications of an infection on July 15, 1940.

Services were held at the Alton funeral home, and it was estimated that more than 46,000 people viewed his body. Robert Wadlow was buried in the Oakwood Cemetery in Upper Alton, Illinois. His coffin measured 10 feet, 9 inches (328 cm) long and weighed over 1,000 pounds (453.6 kg). Before Wadlow died, he heard stories about physicians and anatomical museums that collected the remains of giants and other human oddities. He begged his parents not to let that happen to him. At Wadlow's request, his family placed his coffin in a protective casing of reinforced concrete to protect his remains from curiosity seekers. For this reason, his family also destroyed most of his belongings, not wanting collectors to obtain his clothes or personal items.[10] To this day, he remains an honored part of Illinois history at the Alton Museum of History and Art, where a life-size statue of the town's native son has stood since 1985.

---

9  "Charles A. Leone, "The Story of Robert," Carlton TV, London, 1975, https://www.youtube.com/watch?v=fQHI15sUDjE.

10  Frederick Drimmer, *Born Different: Amazing Stories of Very Special People* (New York: Bantam Skylark Book, 1991), 70-71.

# CHAPTER 13

# THE FUTURE

By the time I met them, Brendan and Professor Korbonits had known each other for more than ten years and had discussed and gathered information in hopes that one day a book about Irish giants would be written. After I met Brendan and we decided to team up to create this book, it was nice to find out that I was a bit of serendipity in his life. He long believed that given the Great Famine and the colonization of Ireland that drove the Irish from their homeland out into the world, there had to be others with gigantism related to their Irish roots living in the United States and beyond. I was Brendan's proof that he was right.

I may have been the first to be identified with the genetic mutation, but I am certainly not the only one. There must be others in the United States and in other countries such as Canada and Australia where the Irish diaspora fled. Our hope is that this book will find its way into their hands and lead them to the medical support they need for themselves and their families.

While writing this book, I quickly learned that every answer to one of my questions about genetic gigantism only led to more questions. I realized that researchers experience the same situation. The more they answer questions, the more questions appear, pulling their research forward into the future. So, what does the future hold for researchers engaged in studying rare diseases, such as genetic gigantism?

Professor Korbonits pointed out that the future depends on the dedication and tenacity of a new generation of talented researchers who are developing their own research projects. I was fortunate that one of those very talented researchers, Dr. Ben Loughrey, was already involved in this book project. We met up with him when I was in London, and I talked with him several times over the past year when he joined in on some of our Zoom calls. I called on him to help me see into the future of genetic gigantism research. We started by discussing the challenges researchers face.

Dr. Loughrey pointed out that the first challenge is simply finding patients with acromegaly or gigantism, given the difficulty patients report in getting a diagnosis for such a rare disease. "I have the data on all different types of pituitary tumors, not just ones that cause acromegaly or gigantism, where the patients are from in Northern Ireland, and what medical specialty or surgery they've come from. These people come through all kinds of services before they're diagnosed, including orthopedics, rheumatology, neurology, ophthalmology, and dermatology. They are lucky that they finally get diagnosed, but they should have been that lucky five or ten years before."

I asked him to give me some examples. "One person was just out walking, and a nurse stopped him and told him that he had acromegaly and that he needed to see a doctor. Another person happened to be in the waiting area with their friend who was the one scheduled to see the endocrinologist for a thyroid problem. When the person came into the clinic room with their friend, the endocrinologist asked him if he had ever been told he had acromegaly." As it turned out, the endocrinologist's observation was correct. Simply by noticing the physical characteristics of acromegaly, the doctor helped him get the treatment he needed.

Getting a correct diagnosis for a rare disease leading to an effective treatment plan is difficult for anyone with a rare disease. According to both the US Genetic and Rare Diseases Information Center and the UK Rare Diseases Framework, there are more than 10,000 rare diseases. While each individual disease may be exceedingly rare, more than 30 million patients in the US and 3.5 million in the UK experience a rare disease. The average time to diagnosis is more than four years. Many take much longer and require extensive testing and evaluation before a treatment plan can be developed. The disease may be rare, but the diagnostic odyssey is not.

Dr. Loughrey's comments turned to another challenge. "There is this suspicion or mystery around medical research. I have seen patients with pituitary conditions and offered to involve them in pituitary research. We would have a chat, and I'd leave them information sheets and consent forms to allow us to enter their data into Professor Korbonits' database anonymously. When I returned, patients often expressed concern about data and privacy. These are legitimate concerns, and I try to put their mind at ease, but in some instances, they aren't confident in the research infrastructure." Despite rigorous safeguards to protect patient data and anonymity, it remains a challenge to assure patients of confidentiality.

I knew from talking with him previously that gathering consent forms, tracking patients, and inputting data was a very time-consuming yet vital part of his research. I asked him how he coped. "There is a vocation in it. There's an element of just being stubborn and tenacious. Now that I am in clinic, the local physicians know that I've got a very niche interest in this topic and am very keen to talk with anybody with the *AIP* variant or who is very young with acromegaly. I am constantly keeping my ear to the ground. I get the neurosurgical list every week for pituitary surgeries, and I database every surgery anonymously. If someone has acromegaly, I ask when it started and what part of Northern Ireland they are from. Right now, I am in a clinic with lots of other practitioners, but my hope is one day to have my own clinic. Maybe I'll be known as the guy with an interest in this, and patients will get referred and come my way naturally." Despite the challenges, Dr. Loughrey was clear in his commitment to the field of genetic studies by staying vigilant in contacting patients who may be at risk and stalwart in maintaining the confidentiality and security of any medical data derived from patients.

Our discussion turned to the future. What is on the horizon for researchers? His response was hopeful. "One of the exciting things in the future for those with the *AIP* variant is that we eventually should under-stand who is more likely to develop the pituitary tumor. I think we will be able to do that in the future, and it is more of a question of when and how than if." Even though it is a rare disease, there are over 200 people in the database, and Professor Korbonits' group is using the blood samples to compare who developed the condition versus people who didn't develop the condition.

Dr. Loughrey noted that it is very challenging for physicians to keep up with all the research being done in genetics and rare diseases. "Things are very dynamic these days from a genetics perspective. Despite the difficulty, you need to stay up to date, particularly with rare diseases. Any potential to identify a rare disease early is extremely important." It is critical for patients to know as soon as possible that they have a rare disease, so researchers aim to be proactive not reactive.

To that end, another positive sign for the future of rare genetic disorders is the creation of genome projects that focus on testing newborns for genetic diseases. The United Kingdom, for example, recently launched a whole-genome sequencing program with the goal of sequencing the genomes of 100,000 newborn babies.[1] The hope is to detect 200 rare but treatable genetic conditions, eliminating the diagnostic odyssey so common in rare disorders. Not only will families and their newborns potentially be spared the pain and suffering from a long-delayed diagnosis, but also the healthcare system will benefit from reduced costs by eliminating unnecessary testing that plays a role in the challenge of finding the right diagnosis for a rare disorder.[2]

In the United States, the BabySeq Project, Phase 1 was a first-of-its-kind randomized clinical trial to incorporate genomic sequencing into routine newborn care by building on existing newborn testing.[3] All new-

---

1 Contact https://www.generationstudy.co.uk/ for more information.

2 Thomas Page, "100,000 newborn babies will have their genomes sequenced in the UK. It could have big implications for child medicine," *CNN Health*. https://www.cnn.com/2023/03/19/health/newborn-genomes-programme-uk-genomics-scn-spc-intl/index.html

3 More information at https://www.genomes2people.org/research/babyseq/

borns in the US already have a blood test shortly after birth to screen for around 30 inherited conditions. Newborn genomic sequencing supplements that test, and it screens for thousands of additional disorders that newborns could be at risk for developing during childhood. Preliminary data from the project shows positive results for the earlier diagnosis of genetic conditions without undue psychological stress for parents. Phase 2 of the project is underway with plans to enroll 500 new babies before the project is completed in 2025.

The future is bright due to dedicated researchers studying rare diseases and patients willing to participate in their vital research. There is hope. In a 2015 article, Professor Korbonits underscored the goal of her research into the rare disease of genetic gigantism. "Our aim with the genetic studies and studying giants is to identify the families; find the carrier of the gene; and discover who develops the disease and treat them in time, well before they truly develop extreme height and all of the awful complications of this disease....Their final height will actually not be gigantic, and they will have, hopefully, close to normal life expectancy. The motto is 'No more giants.'"[4]

The discovery of the *AIP* mutation, like many other discoveries of genetic mutations, is wondrous. It demands years of research using cutting-edge technology and a dose of serendipity to figure out the complex nature of any aspect of the human genome. It is a testimony to the persistence of researchers who peer into the genome, find the pathological gene, and then link that gene to a specific disease. The benefits of genetic testing for a pathological gene variant are clear. A mysterious medical condition can be revealed for what it is: an illness caused by a faulty gene passed down through generations and across the branches of a family tree. Not all cases of gigantism have been linked to a genetic mutation,

---

4 Márta Korbonits, MD, PhD, "Research Goal: 'No More Giants,'" *Medscape*, published April 24, 2015, https://www.medscape.com/viewarticle/843414?form=fpf.

but for those cases that have been, gigantism is no longer simply a matter of myth popping up for no apparent reason with no hope of controlling its consequences.

Having a rare disease can be overwhelming. Simply getting a diagnosis can be a quest through many branches of medicine, leading to an uncertain future. As researchers follow genetic patterns through multiple generations in a family, there is also hope that scientists can find genes related to other rare diseases and give families the tools they need to manage a disease found in their family tree. Brendan and I want all patients with a rare disease to know that they are not alone. We may not share the same rare disease as you do, but we understand what it is like to be isolated by a medical condition that is not easily recognized or understood. We may not be kin, but we are kindred spirits as we travel through our medical journeys—separate but not alone.

# ACKNOWLEDGEMENTS

rendan and I would like to express our deepest gratitude to Professor Márta Korbonits for her unfailing support of this book project. I will never forget the first time I encountered Professor Korbonits when I emailed her over three years ago. Not only did she email me right back despite the late hour, but she also signed her name in an unexpected way. Márta. Simply Márta. I knew from that moment that she was an ally, not just to me but to all her patients who have benefitted from her research and clinical practice.

We would like to thank Professor Mike Besser and Dr. Ben Loughrey for their expertise and kindness as well as the scientists, researchers, and clinicians of St. Bartholomew's Hospital who exemplify Barts' 900 years of compassionate care. Many others have contributed in some way to the creation of this book, including Dr. Mária Hérincs-Whitehead, Aidan Holland, Julian Fowler, Will Palin, Jonathan Gray, Dr. Cecilia Ward, Rita Kelly McCaughey, and Anne McAllister. Brendan thanks his wife Patricia and his sons Stephen and Micheal Holland for their love and support.

This book would not have been possible without my newfound relatives, Niamh Feeney, Laura Holland Jackson, and Phil Burnside, who patiently answered my questions about their medical odyssey. I am also grateful to filmmaker Ronan McCloskey for his encouragement and support and his compassionate portrayal of my cousin Charles Byrne.

I want to thank Suzi Gillette for believing in me from the very beginning and reading my early drafts, editor Tamela Rich for helping me make "book magic," and Carla King of Destination Published for giving me the confidence to publish this book. Thank you, Morgan, Wren, Alexander, Emmett, Christina, and Violet, for your support and love. I am lucky to have you in my life.

My computer was a trusted friend through the pandemic, opening the door to not only the world of gigantism but also to online archives and libraries that formed the backbone of my research. I spent many happy hours delving into the Internet Archives (archive.org), which lived up to its mission of providing "universal access to all knowledge" with its amazing holdings, encompassing more than 44 million print materials, 4.8 million images, and 835 billion web pages in its Wayback Machine.

Shortly after I found out that I had the genetic mutation, I started to take Irish classes, at first, to avoid embarrassment when I tried to pronounce the Irish words that I encountered during my research. However, I soon realized that the Irish language is a gateway into Ireland's history and culture and a way to better understand the forces that shaped my ancestors and me. I have found a welcome home in the vibrant online community of Irish language speakers, especially with Damian Uí Néill and the teachers of online classes at Cairde Uí Néill in Coalisland and Molly Nic Céile of Gaeilge i mo Chroí who patiently taught me to be brave with my bit of Irish and to speak even when I am afraid.

# RESOURCES

We appreciate your interest in our book and its exploration of genetic gigantism in the north of Ireland and beyond. If you have any questions, comments, or would like to share your own experiences, we invite you to visit our website at www.insearchofgiants.org.

If you would like more in-depth information or if you have specific medical questions or concerns about gigantism and Irish giants, we recommend consulting the website for familial isolated pituitary adenomas (FIPA) at Queen Mary University of London. This website is a valuable source of current research, expert insights, and additional support for those interested in exploring this topic further. The website can be found at www.qmul.ac.uk/fipa-patients.

The FIPA website was organized by Professor Korbonits' clinical group in the Department of Endocrinology at St. Bartholomew's Hospital in London in collaboration with the International FIPA Consortium. The Consortium, which started in 2006, is made up of doctors, clinicians, and researchers from around the world, including the United States, Italy, Romania, Australia, and Brazil who care for patients with a range of conditions related to familial isolated pituitary adenomas.

The pituitary tumor, or adenoma, that results in genetic gigantism, as discussed in this book, is a type of familial isolated pituitary adenoma. FIPA is defined as a rare genetic condition characterized by the occurrence of noncancerous pituitary tumors in multiple family members without other related conditions or tumors. There are other disorders besides gigantism caused by having FIPA, and the Queen Mary University of London website is an excellent resource to learn about all types.

Please note that these recommendations do not substitute for professional medical advice, and you are encouraged to consult with your healthcare providers for personalized guidance.

# GLOSSARY

**Acromegaly**: A rare hormonal disorder that occurs when the pituitary gland produces excessive growth hormone. This excess hormone leads to the enlargement of bones and tissues, particularly in the hands, feet, and face.

**Adenoma**: A noncancerous tumor that forms in glandular tissues.

*AIP* (**Aryl hydrocarbon receptor interacting protein**): A molecule that interacts with the aryl hydrocarbon receptor (AhR) and is associated with regulating pituitary cell functions as well as other cellular functions.

**Benign tumor**: A noncancerous growth of cells that does not invade nearby tissues or spread to other parts of the body.

**Carpal Tunnel Syndrome**: A condition where there is pressure on the median nerve as it passes through a narrow passage called the carpal tunnel in the wrist, resulting in numbness, tingling, or weakness in the hand and fingers.

**DNA** (**deoxyribonucleic acid**): A molecule that contains genetic information and instructions for protein synthesis used in the development, functioning, growth, and reproduction of living organisms.

**Endocrine system**: A complex network of glands that produce and release chemical messengers, or hormones, which regulate physiological functions in the body.

**Endocrinologist**: A medical doctor who specializes in diagnosing and treating disorders related to the endocrine system.

**FIPA (Familial isolated pituitary adenoma)**: A rare genetic condition characterized by the occurrence of noncancerous pituitary tumors in multiple family members without other related features or tumors.

**Familial disease**: A genetic disease which runs in a family due to a change in the family's DNA.

**Gene**: A segment of DNA, located on a chromosome, which carries the instructions for making a specific protein or RNA molecule and plays a fundamental role in determining the traits and characteristics of an organism.

**Gene mutation**: A permanent alteration in the DNA sequence of a gene, which can happen spontaneously or due to external factors such as radiation or exposure to chemicals. Some mutations have no noticeable effect while others can contribute to genetic disorders or play a role in diseases.

**Gene variant**: A specific version of a gene. Gene variation is common and considered normal. Some genetic variation, however, can be associated with specific traits, conditions, or diseases.

**Geneticist**: A doctor who specializes in the diagnosis and counseling of patients with hereditary or familial diseases.

**Genome**: The complete set of genes or genetic material present in a cell or organism, containing all the information needed for an organism to develop and function.

**Gigantism/giantism/pituitary acromegaly**: A condition caused by the production of too much growth hormone during childhood or adolescence that occurs before the growth plates of the bones, or epiphyses, have fused.

**Growth hormone**: A hormone produced by the pituitary gland which promotes bone and tissue growth in childhood and adolescence and plays a role in cell reproduction and metabolic regulation in adulthood.

**Hormone**: A chemical messenger produced by glands in the endocrine system and released into the bloodstream to regulate physiological functions.

**Lanreotide**: A somatostatin analogue used to reduce levels of growth hormone.

**Microsatellites**: Short, repeated sequences of DNA found along a chromosome.

**Mid-parental height**: An estimate of how tall a child is likely to be as an adult, based on the average height of their biological parents with adjustments made for gender differences.

**Pituitary apoplexy**: A rare but serious condition that occurs when there is bleeding or impaired blood flow to the pituitary gland.

**Pituitary fossa**: The bony pocket in the skull where the pituitary gland is located.

**Pituitary gland**: A small, pea-sized gland, which is located at the base of the brain within a bony structure called the pituitary fossa, which plays a central role in regulating physiological processes by producing and releasing hormones.

**Pituitary adenoma**: A noncancerous tumor that develops in the pituitary gland.

**Penetrance**: The proportion of individuals with a disease-causing mutation who exhibit clinical symptoms.

**Prevalence**: The frequency or occurrence of a specific genetic trait, condition, or variation within a population.

**Prolactinoma**: A noncancerous tumor of the pituitary gland that results in the overproduction of prolactin, a hormone known for its role in enabling mammals to produce milk.

**Radiotherapy**: A medical treatment that uses high-dose radiation to shrink tumors and prevent their growth.

**Transsphenoidal surgery**: A procedure used to remove tumors or lesions near the pituitary gland by making a small incision inside the nostril or upper gum to access the pituitary gland through the sphenoid sinus.

**Visual field test**: A diagnostic test measuring the extent of peripheral vision, which is the ability to see objects and movement outside the direct line of sight.

# BIBLIOGRAPHY

Acosta, Joseph de. *History of the Indies, Vol. II.* Translated by Edward Grimston. New York: Burt Franklin, 1970. Originally published 1590.

Altick, Richard D. *The Shows of London.* Cambridge, MA: Harvard University Press, 1978.

Armocida, Emanuele, Raffaella Bianucci, Elena Varotto, W.W. de Herder, and Francesco M. Galassi, "Hereditary acromegalic gigantism in the family of Roman Emperor Maximinus Thrax," *Medical Hypotheses* 136 (2020): 109525.

Ball, James Moores. *The Body Snatchers.* New York: Dorset Press, 1928.

Beckers, Albert, Maya Beth Lodish, Giampaolo Trivellin, Liliya Rostomyan, Misu Lee, Fabio R. Faucz, Bo Yuan, Catherine S. Choong, Jean-Hubert Caberg, Elisa Verrua, Luciana Ansaneli Naves, Tim D. Cheetham, Jacques Young, Philippe A. Lys, Patrick Petrossians, Andrew Cotterill, Nalini Samir Sha, Daniel Metzger, Emilie Castermans, Maria Rosaria Ambrosi, Chiara Villa, Natalia Strebkova, Nadia Mazerkina, Stéphan Gaillarda, Gustavo Barcelos Barr, Luis Augusto Casulari, Sebastian J. Neggers, Roberto Salvatori, Marie-Lise Jaffrain-Rea, Margaret Zacharin, Beatriz Lecumberri Santamaria, Sabina Zachariev, Ee Mun Lim, Giovanna Mantovani, Maria Chiara Zatelli, Michael T. Collins, Jean-François Bonneville, Martha Quezado, Prashant Chittiboina, Edward H. Oldfield, Vincent Bour, Pengfei Liu, Wouter W. de Herder, Natalia Pellegata, James R. Lupski, Adrian F. Daly, and Constantine A. Stratakis. "X-linked acrogigantism syndrome: clinical profile and therapeutic responses." *Endocrine-Related Cancer* 22, no. 3 (2015): 353-367.

Boguszewski, Cesar Luiz, Margaret Cristina da Silva Boguszewski, and Wouter W. de Herder. "From Dwarves to Giants: South American's Contribution to the History of Growth Hormone and Related Disorders." *Growth Hormone & IGF Research* 50 (2020): 48–56.

Chahal, Harvinder S., Karen Stals, Martina Unterländer, David J. Balding, Mark G. Thomas, Ajith V. Kumar, G. Michael Besser, A. Brew Atkinson, Patrick J. Morrison, Trevor A. Howlett, Miles J. Levy, Steve M. Orme, Scott A. Akker, Richard L. Abel, Ashley B. Grossman, Joachim Burger, Sian Ellard, and Márta Korbonits. "*AIP* Mutation in Pituitary Adenomas in the 18th Century and Today." *The New England Journal of Medicine* 8 (2011).

"Census 2022: Ireland's population hits record levels." *BBC News*, June 23, 2022, www.bbc.com/news/uk-northern-ireland-61910927. Accessed October 30, 2023.

Cubbage, Eric. "The Tragic Story of Charles Byrne 'The Irish Giant'." Web archive. http://www.thetallestman.com/pdf/charlesbyrne.pdf. Accessed September 7, 2023.

de Herder, Wouter W. "4 Movie Actors with Acromegaly/Gigantism." *Journal of Endocrinological Investigation* 32 (2009): 791–792.

de Herder, Wouter W. "Acromegalic Gigantism, Physicians and Body Snatching: Past or Present?." *Pituitary* 15, no. 3 (2012): 312.

de Herder, Wouter W. "Acromegaly and Gigantism in the Medical Literature. Case Descriptions in the Era Before and the Early Years After the Initial Publication of Pierre Marie (1886)." *Pituitary* 12 (2009): 236–244.

de Herder, Wouter W. "Aldo Molinari: The Wedding of the Giant Almiro Crema in Torino." *Journal of Endocrinological Investigation* 45 (2022): 1117–1120.

de Herder, Wouter W. "Familial Gigantism." *Clinics* 67 (2012): 29–32.

de Herder, Wouter W. "The History of Acromegaly." *Neuroendocrinology* 103 (2016): 7–17.

Donnelly, Deidre E. and Patrick J. Morrison. "Hereditary Gigantism – The Biblical Giant Goliath and His Brothers." *The Ulster Medical Journal*, 83, no. 2 (May 1, 2014): 86-88.

Drimmer, Frederick. *Born Different: Amazing Stories of Very Special People*. New York: Bantam Skylark Book, 1991.

Fowler, Julian. "Acromegaly: 'Giant gene' bond forged between Us and Mid Ulster." *BBC Northern Ireland*. June 8, 2022. www.bbc.com/news/uk-northern-ireland-61726811. Accessed October 29, 2023.

Fowler, Julian. "Land of the Giants?" *BBC News*. February 8, 2013. https://www.bbc.com/news/av/uk-northern-ireland-21387358. Accessed January 24, 2024.

Frankcom, Graham and Jonathan H. Musgrave. *The Irish Giant*. London: Gerald Duckworth & Co., 1976.

Frazer, William, and G. Henry Kinahan. "Giant's Grave, Loughry Demesne, County Tyrone." National Library of Ireland, Sketch Books of Irish Antiquities. Catalogue No. PD 1975 TX 27 (29). https://catalogue.nli.ie/Record/vtls000745296/HoldingsILS#tabnav.

Gadelha, Monica R., Toni R. Prezant, Karina N. Une, Roberta P. Glick, Stanley F. Moskal, II, Mario Vaisman, Shlomo Melmed, Rhonda D. Kineman, and Lawrence A. Frohman, "Loss of Heterozygosity on Chromosome 11q13 in Two Families with Acromegaly/Gigantism Is Independent of Mutations of the Multiple Endocrine Neoplasia Type I Gene." *Journal of Clinical Endocrinology and Metabolism* 84 (1999): 249-256.

Igaz, Peter and Attila Patócs, eds. *Genetics of Endocrine Diseases and Syndromes*. Vol. 111. Springer International Publishing, 2019.

*Gentleman's Magazine.* 53 (1783): 541.

"Irish Place Names," *Tailte Éireann*, osi.ie/blog/irish-place-names. Accessed April 26, 2023.

Jennings, Juliet E., Marianthi Georgitsi, Ian Holdaway, Adrian F Daly, Maria Tichomirowa, Albert Beckers, Lauri A. Aaltonen, Auli Karhu, and Fergus J Cameron. "Aggressive Pituitary Adenomas Occurring in Young Patients in a Large Polynesian Kindred with a Germline R271W Mutation in the *AIP* Gene." *European Journal of Endocrinology* 161 (2009): 799–804.

Johnson, Ben. "The Reputed Plague Pits of London." *Historic UK.* https://www.historic-uk.com/HistoryMagazine/DestinationsUK/LondonPlaguePits/. Accessed October 2, 2023.

Kobler, John. *The Reluctant Surgeon: A Biography of John Hunter.* New York: Akadine Press, 1999.

Korbonits, Márta. "Ghrelin—a hormone with multiple functions." *Frontiers in Neuroendocrinology* 25, no. 1 (April 2004): 27-68.

Korbonits, Márta. "Research Goal: 'No More Giants.'" *Medscape.* April 24, 2015. https://www.medscape.com/viewarticle/843414?form=fpf. Accessed November 11, 2023.

Landolt, A.M., and Zachmann, M. "The Irish Giant: New Observations Concerning the Nature of His Ailment." *Lancet* 1, no. 8181 (1980): 1311-1312.

Leone, Charles A., "The Story of Robert." *Carlton TV*, London, 1975. https://www.youtube.com/watch?v=fQHI15sUDjE. Accessed September 8, 2023.

Loughrey, Paul Benjamin and Márta Korbonits. "Genetics of Pituitary Tumors," in *Genetics of Endocrine Diseases and Syndromes*, eds. Peter Igaz and Attila Patócs, 171-212. Springer International Publishing, 2019.

Markantes, Georgios K., Anastasia Theodoropoulou, Anastasia K. Armeni, Vasiliki Vasileiou, Constantine A. Stratakis, and Neoklis A. Georgopoulos. "Cyclopes and Giants: From Homer's Odyssey to Contemporary Genetic Diagnosis." *Hormones* 15, no. 3 (2016):459-463.

Marques, Pedro, Francisca Caimari, Laura C. Hernández-Ramírez, Avid Collier, Donato Iacovazzo, Amy Ronaldson, Kesson Magid, Chung Thong Lim, Karen Stals, Sian Ellard, Ashley B. Grossman, and Márta Korbonits. "Significant Benefits of *AIP* Testing and Clinical Screening in Familial Isolated and Young-onset Pituitary Tumors." *Journal of Clinical Endocrinology and Metabolism* 105, no. 6 (2020): e2247–60.

McCarron, Edward T. "Altered States: Tyrone Migration to Providence, Rhode Island During the Nineteenth Century." *Clogher Record* vol. 16, no. 1 (1997): 145-161.

McCloskey, Ronan. *Charles Byrne: the Irish Giant/an Fathach Éireannach*. Directed by Ronan McCloskey. BBC Northern Ireland, 2011. https://www.youtube.com/watch?v=xLA-KZ7sBLg. Accessed June 22, 2024.

McCorristine, Shane. "The Dark Value of Criminal Bodies: Context, Consent, and the Disturbing Sale of John Parker's Skull." *Journal of Conservation and Museum Studies* 13 (2015).

Miller, Kerby. *Emigrants and Exiles: Ireland and the Irish Exodus to North America*. New York: Oxford University Press, 1985.

Mills, Georgia. "Hormones: The Inside Story, Episode 7 – Will taking hormones make me taller?" *Society for Endocrinology*: https://www.yourhormones.info/resources/digital-library/podcasts/will-taking-hormones-make-me-taller/#:~:text=If%20you're%20an%20adult,answer%20is%20a%20definitive%20no. Accessed October 26, 2023.

Minozzi, Simona, Walter Pantano, Francesco di Gennaro, Gino Fornaciari, and Paola Catalano. "Pituitary Disease from the Past: A Rare Case of Gigantism in Skeletal Remains from the Roman Imperial Age." *The Journal of Clinical Endocrinology & Metabolism* 97 (2012): 4302–4303.

Moore, Wendy. *The Knife Man: Blood, Body Snatching, and the Birth of Modern Surgery.* New York: Broadway Books, 2005.

Morley, Henry. *Memoirs of Bartholomew Fairs*, originally published in 1857. George Routledge and Sons, London, 1892.

Muinzer, Thomas L. "A Grave Situation: An Examination of the Legal Issues Raised by the Life and Death of Charles Byrne, the 'Irish Giant'." *International Journal of Cultural Property* 20 (2013): 23–48.

Mulvihill, Jerry. *The Truth about the Irish Famine 1845-1852.* 2020.

Nash, Catherine. "Making Kinship with Human Remains: Repatriation, Biomedicine and the Many Relations of Charles Byrne." *Environment and Planning D: Society and Space* 36 (2018): 867–884.

National Folklore Collection, University College Dublin. "The Schools' Collection." www.duchas.ie/en/cbes. Accessed January 24, 2024.

*Ordnance Survey Memoirs of Ireland: Parishes of Co. Londonderry 1, 1830, 1834, 1836*, edited by Angelique Day and Patrick McWilliams. Institute of Irish, 1990.

Ó Tuathail, Eámonn. *Sgéalta Mhuintir Luinigh: Munterloney Folktales: Irish Traditions from County Tyrone.* Folklore of Ireland Council, 193. Reprint, 2015.

Page, Thomas. "100,000 newborn babies will have their genomes sequenced in the UK. It could have big implications for child medicine." *CNN Health.* https://www.cnn.com/2023/03/19/health/newborn-genomes-programme-uk-genomics-scn-spc-intl/index.html. Accessed November 11, 2023.

Prezio, Joseph. A., Joseph E. Griffin, and John J. O'Brien. "Acromegalic Gigantism: The Buffalo Giant." *The American Journal of Medicine* 31 (1961): 966–976.

"Public Health Challenges of Disease." *National Institutes of Health, Genetic and Rare Diseases Information Center.* https://rarediseases.info.nih.gov/. Accessed October 23, 2023.

Radian, Serban, Yoan Diekmann, Plamena Gabrovska, Brendan Holland, Lisa Bradley, Helen Wallace, Karen Stals, Anna-Marie Bussell, Karen McGurren, Martin Cuesta, Anthony W. Ryan, Maria Herincs, Laura C. Hernández-Ramírez, Aidan Holland, Jade Samuels, Elena Daniela Aflorei, Sayka Barry, Judit Dénes, Ida Pernicova, Craig E. Stiles, Giampaolo Trivellin, Ronan McCloskey, Michal Ajzensztejn, Noina Abid, Scott A. Akker, Moises Mercado, Mark Cohen, Rajesh V. Thakker, Stephanie Baldeweg, Ariel Barkan, Madalina Musat, Miles Levy, Stephen M. Orme, Martina Unterländer, Joachim Burger, Ajith V. Kumar, Sian Ellard, Joseph McPartlin, Ross McManus, Gerard J. Linden, Brew Atkinson, David J. Balding, Amar Agha, Chris J. Thompson, Steven J. Hunter, Mark G. Thomas, Patrick J. Morrison, and Márta Korbonits. "Increased Population Risk of *AIP*-Related Acromegaly and Gigantism in Ireland." *Human Mutation* 38 (2017): 78-85.

Radian, Serban and Maria Herincs. "Legends And Facts: Population Screening for *AIP* Mutations in Northern Ireland." *The Endocrinologist* Summer 2013: 24-25.

Ramírez-Rentería, Claudia, Laura C. Hernández-Ramírez, Lesly Portocarrero-Ortiz, Guadalupe Vargas, Virgilio Melgar, Etual Espinosa, Ana Laura Espinosa-de-los-Monteros, Ernesto Sosa, Baldomero González, Sergio Zúñiga, Martina Unterländer, Joachim Burger, Karen Stals, Anne-Marie Bussell, Sian Ellard, Mary Dang, Donato Iacovazzo, Sonal Kapur, Plamena Gabrovska, Serban Radian, Federico Roncaroli, Márta Korbonits and Moisés Mercado. "*AIP* mutations in young patients with acromegaly and the Tampico Giant: the Mexican experience." *Endocrine Genetics/Epigenetics* 53, no. 3 (2016): 402-411.

Rumsey, Nichola. "Body Image and Congenital Conditions with Visible Differences." In *Body Image: A Handbook of Theory, Research, and Clinical Practice*, edited by Thomas F. Cash and Thomas Pruzinsky, 229. New York: The Guilford Press, 2002.

Soares, Beatriz S., Kuniki Eguchi, and Lawrence A. Frohman. "Tumor deletion mapping on chromosome 11q13 in eight families with isolated familial somatotropinoma and in 15 sporadic somatotropinomas." *Journal of Clinical Endocrinology and Metabolism* 90, no. 12 (2005): 6580-6587.

Takada, Kazuhide, Mari Sasano, and Satoshi Hayakawa."A Legendary Sumo Wrestler with Gigantism or Acromegaly? The Case of Ikezuki Geitazaemon (1827–1850)." *Medical Hypotheses* 144 (2020): 110174.

*The Morning Herald*, 6 May 1782.

The Royal Colleges of Surgeons, Society for Endocrinology. "A Tall Story: Unravelling the Genetics Behind Charles Byrne – 'The Irish Giant.'" Video. London, November 23, 2011. https://youtu.be/IWaPgnk1-Kc. Accessed January 24, 2024.

*The Town and Country Magazine, Or, Universal Repository of Knowledge, Instruction, and Entertainment*: Volume 14, August 1782.

"The UK Rare Diseases Framework" *United Kingdom Department of Health & Social Care*. https://www.gov.uk/government/publications/uk-rare-diseases-framework/the-uk-rare-diseases-framework. Accessed October 23, 2023.

*True North: The Giant Gene*. Directed by Chris Nikkel. BBC One Northern Ireland, June 18, 2018.

Ua Cróinín, Risteard. Clare County Library. "Importance of Placenames." www.clarelibrary.ie/eolas/coclare/places/importance_of_placenames.htm. Accessed January 24, 2024.

"Väinö Myllyrinne le géant finnois." July 29, 1935. https://www.youtube.com/watch?v=U_qjXt9T3kQ. Accessed January 24, 2024.

Vierimaa, Outi, Marianthi Georgitsi, Rainer Lehtonen, Pia Vahteristo, Antti Kokko, Anniina Raitila, Karoliina Tuppurainen, Tapani M. L. Ebeling, Pasi I. Salmela, Ralf Paschke, Sadi Gündogdu, Ernesto De Menis, Markus J. Mäkinen, Virpi Launonen, Auli Karhu, and Lauri A. Aaltonen "Pituitary adenoma predisposition caused by germline mutations in the *AIP* gene." *Science* 312, no. 5777 (May 26, 2006): 1228-1230.

Williams, Fred, Steven Hunter, Lisa Bradley, Harvinder S. Chahal, Helen L. Storr, Scott A. Akker, Ajith V. Kumar, Stephen M. Orme, Jane Evanson, Noina Abid, Patrick J. Morrison, Márta Korbonits, and A. Brew Atkinson "Clinical Experience in the Screening and Management of a Large Kindred with Familial Isolated Pituitary Adenoma Due to an Aryl Hydrocarbon Receptor Interacting Protein (*AIP*) Mutation." *Journal of Clinical Endocrinology & Metabolism* 99, no. 4 (2014): 1122-1131.

Wood, Edward J. *Giants and Dwarfs.* London: Richard Bentley, 1868.

# IMAGE CREDITS

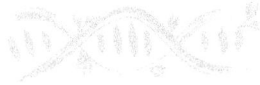

"Round His Head Shone the Red Light" from Heroes of the Dawn by Violet Russell, Illustrated by Beatrice Elvery. Public Domain.

"Woman with Acromegaly," Author unknown. Public Domain.

"A nightwatchman disturbs a body-snatcher who has dropped the stolen corpse he had been carrying in a hamper, while the anatomist runs away." Etching with engraving by W. Austin, 1773. Wellcome Collection. Attribution 4.0 International (CC BY 4.0).

"Two men placing the shrouded corpse which they have just disinterred into a sack while Death, as a nightwatchman holding a lantern, grabs one of the grave-robbers from behind." Coloured drawing by T. Rowlandson, 1775. Wellcome Collection. Public Domain.

"Charles Byrne, a giant, George Cranstoun, a dwarf, and three other normal sized men." Etching by J. Kay, 1794. Wellcome Collection. Public Domain.

"Three anatomical dissections taking place in an attic." Coloured lithograph by T. C. Wilson after a pen and wash drawing by T. Rowlandson. Wellcome Collection. Public Domain.

"Three giants, the tallest identified as Charles Byrne and the others as twins, and six spectators including an unidentified lady and dwarf." Etching by J. Kay, 1784, after himself. Wellcome Collection. Public Domain.

"Robert Wadlow and his father," postcard created 1937. Photographer unknown. Public Domain.

All other photographs or images used with the permission of the owners.

# ABOUT THE AUTHORS

**COLLEEN SNYDER**, MA in Literature and Language,
**The American University, Washington, D.C.**
Colleen lives in the Blue Ridge Mountains of Virginia. In 2020, she discovered that she had a rare *AIP* genetic mutation normally found in Northern Ireland that caused her childhood-onset acromegalic gigantism. Knowing that her ancestors came from that area in 1861, she contacted London physician Professor Márta Korbonits about her work with patients from Northern Ireland. Professor Korbonits told her that she was the first person in the United Stated identified with the Irish variant and introduced her to Brendan who has the same genetic mutation and shares her diagnosis of gigantism. A former college writing teacher, Colleen has been published in *The Washington Post* and *Destinations* magazine.

**BRENDAN HOLLAND**, Joint Honorable President and Committee
**Member of the Killeeshil & Clonaneese Historical Society in Dungannon,**
**County Tyrone, Northern Ireland, United Kingdom**
Brendan has lived most of his life in the Dungannon area which is part of the geographic hotspot for the *AIP* mutation found in Northern Ireland identified through Professor Korbonits' research. In 2009, he met Professor Korbonits during the filming of the documentary *Charles Byrne, the Irish Giant* directed by Ronan McCloskey in which Brendan played a prominent role. Brendan was also featured in the 2016 BBC documentary *The Giant Gene*. He has researched the history of gigantism in the geographic hotspot and has been interviewed on the NBC Today Show, BBC Radio 4, Irish Examiner, RTE Radio 1, and the BBC World Service.